W9-BPL-529

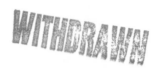
WITHDRAWN

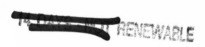

Hepatitis B

Baruch S. Blumberg

Hepatitis B

THE HUNT FOR A KILLER VIRUS

PRINCETON UNIVERSITY PRESS

PRINCETON AND OXFORD

Published by Princeton University Press, 41 William Street, Princeton, New Jersey 08540

In the United Kingdom: Princeton University Press, 3 Market Place, Woodstock, Oxfordshire OX20 1SY

Library of Congress Cataloging-in-Publication Data

Blumberg, Baruch S., 1925–

Hepatitis B : the hunt for a killer virus / Baruch S. Blumberg.

p. cm.

Includes bibliographical references and index.

ISBN 0-691-00692-X (alk. paper)

1. Hepatitis B virus—Research—History. 2. Hepatitis B vaccine—Research—History. I. Title.

QR201.H46 B58 2001

616.3'6230194—dc21   2001051361

British Library Cataloging-in-Publication Data is available

This book has been composed in Palatino and Helvetica Neue by Gary R. Beck

Printed on acid-free paper ∞

www.pup.princeton.edu

Printed in the United States of America

1 2 3 4 5 6 7 8 9 10

*T*o Jean

My wife, Jean, maintained the normalcy and steadiness of our family that has balanced a life that could easily have been caught up in the whirlwinds of action and imagination swirling through the world of the scientist. We have shared love, friendship, children, and grandchildren together for many decades. I could not have accomplished the work described in this book without her.

And to Miriam Fischman

Miriam, my sister, has been a steadfast friend who has become the center of our small extended family. She has had more of an influence on my life than I think she knows.

Suppose he'd listened to the erudite committee,
He only would have found where not to look;
Suppose his terrier when he whistled had obeyed,
It would not have unearthed the buried city;
Suppose he had dismissed the careless maid,
The cryptogram would not have fluttered from the book.

—W. H. Auden, "The Quest," 1940

Something hidden. Go and find it. Go and look behind the Ranges—
Something lost behind the Ranges. Lost and waiting for you. Go!

—Rudyard Kipling, "The Explorer," 1898

Contents

Acknowledgments

IN THIS BOOK I describe a phase of the research on hepatitis B virus that my colleagues and I at Fox Chase Cancer Center (and elsewhere) were engaged in over the course of several decades. There were many scientists in other laboratories and clinics who labored in this field of research preceding, during, and after we made our contributions. I am indebted to them for the vast store of knowledge they accumulated that allowed our own research to go forward.

I have been fortunate in having inspiring mentors during my clinical and research training, several of whom are referred to in the text. They were wonderful guides to an often perplexed student, and I greatly appreciate their support of and confidence in their student.

I was an investigator at the National Institutes of Health in Bethesda, Maryland, during the early part of the research. It was, and is, a remarkable scientific institution that has been responsible in large part for the great advances in medicine in the United States in the last half-century. I am particularly indebted to Dr. Thomas Dublin for making it possible for me to follow a line of research that did not seem, to others, as promising then as it did later. I worked at Fox Chase Cancer Center in Philadelphia for most of my scientific career. It was an ideal environment in which to pursue the curiosity-driven basic research required for our discovery program. Timothy Talbot, who appointed me to the Center, was a remarkable director who taught me most of what I know about the appropriate governance of an institution. He knew when to get out of the way (which was most of the time) and when to provide support. He was also a great friend; all of us at the Center appreciated his principled good sense and wise counsel. Academic institutions are often the scene of battles between the scientific staff and the administration. That was not the case at our Center; Francis McKay and after him Donald Leedy seemed to understand that the administration was supposed to serve the needs of the scientific staff, and they did so very effectively. Little of the research could have been accomplished without my scientific and other colleagues at Fox Chase Cancer Center, and the National Institutes of Health. There would not have been a book without them. I will say more about them in the text and in Appendix 1. Anna Dortort, my secretary at Fox Chase, assisted greatly in the early drafts of this book, as did Maureen Climaldi and Joyce Codispoti. They also provided needed encouragement when my enthusiasm for writing flagged, as it did more frequently than I care to remember.

A large part of this book was written in Stanford, California, when I was a visitor and later a Fellow at the Center for Advanced Study in the Behavioral Studies. It is an ideal venue for thinking and writing, an island of calm and a place for reflection perched on a hillside above the Stanford University campus, overlooking the hectic activity of Silicon Valley. I appreciate the time I spent at the Center and the help I received from the directors and the excellent staff.

The editors at Princeton University Press, particularly Sam Elworthy, were very helpful. Scientific hypotheses and ideas are always subject to refutation; this encourages a tentative sentence structure and the passive voice. Senior editor Lauren Lepow painstakingly copyedited the manuscript and, among other wholesome corrections, changed many of these sentences to the active voice. I appreciate her efforts, and I believe the readers will as well.

The reviewers of the several drafts of this book helped to curb my enthusiasm for too many words, for which I am grateful. My children, Anne, George, Jane, and Noah, provided support and, of course, the usual intergenerational advice. In particular, Jane, a writer herself, read the early manuscripts and provided many useful changes in her attempt to make this book less of a scientific treatise and more of a human document.

Introduction

HEPATITIS B virus (HBV) is one of the most common viruses in the world. Hundreds of millions of people have been infected with it—perhaps half of the world's population—and it ranks as one of the top ten killers of people among the bacteria, protozoans, viruses, parasites, and other infectious agents that plague humankind. The most characteristic clinical sign of hepatitis is the vivid yellow color—jaundice—it imparts to the whites of the eyes and, often, the entire body. Yellow jaundice is the hallmark of the disease and is often the clinical finding that draws attention to the malady, particularly if it occurs in epidemic form. Fortunately, most cases of hepatitis are acute and self-limited, but many progress to a chronic form that can be deadly.

About 1.5 million people worldwide die each year as a consequence of HBV infection. These include about a million people with primary cancer of the liver, one of the most common and deadly cancers known, a large percentage of which are caused by HBV. Currently, over 350 million people are chronically infected with HBV. HBV kills as many, if not more, people than the human immunodeficiency virus (HIV), the deadly causative virus of AIDS.

The presentation of such grim figures as these usually precedes a prediction of even more awful events. But that is not the case for HBV. Life—and death—are full of surprises, and while it may be tempting fate to be too optimistic, it appears likely that within the next few decades this virus will be effectively controlled. It is even possible that it will be eradicated.

Although the diseases associated with yellow jaundice have been recognized since antiquity, the history of research on HBV is not long. The beginning of the "modern" period can be dated to the interval between the two world wars. By the mid-1960s, owing to the efforts of a dedicated and gifted cadre of scientists, there emerged a significant understanding of the clinical and epidemiological nature of the disease, a recognition that it was caused by a "filterable agent"[1]—a virus—and that there were at least two such viruses. In the mid-1960s my colleagues and I in Philadelphia began studies on a material we found in the serum of an Australian, a material that we referred to as "Australia antigen"; by 1967 we had found that it was part of the hepatitis B virus, and we introduced a useful diagnostic method for the virus that, in a relatively short time, essentially eliminated posttransfusion hepatitis due to HBV. In 1969, we invented a vaccine that, in its further development by the pharmaceutical industry, proved to be effective and safe.

Our early work stimulated a worldwide interest in the scientific community, and research in the field proliferated. Today a great deal is known about the virus; effective methods for detection and prevention are available; and there are even reasonably good treatments, along with an expectation that these may improve considerably in the future. As a consequence of the widespread application of the vaccine and other prevention programs, there has been, in several places, a striking decrease in the number of new HBV infections. In parts of Asia, where the vaccine programs were introduced more than ten years ago, the prevalence of carriers with HBV has dropped from about 15 percent to about 1 percent, and, in the impacted vaccinated group, the incidence of cancer of the liver (most of which is caused by chronic HBV infection) has decreased two-thirds from its previous level. If these results are confirmed, then HBV vaccine is the first "cancer vaccine."

Basic research is often *Shandean*, a term coined in the novel *Tristram Shandy* (1759–67) by the Irish-born English writer Laurence

---

[1] The term used for an infectious agent that was known to be smaller than bacteria, and that would pass through a filter too fine to allow the passage of bacteria.

Sterne (1713–68).[2] In this comic novel, any trace of narrative order is subordinated to the free associations generated by the narrator and his characters. Events ramble from one apparent irrelevancy to another, but a strange sense of order nevertheless emerges. The novel also offers an interesting exploration of the quality of time: the description of an event takes far longer than the event itself. For example, the author tells of his own conception but gets so embroiled in the tale of his parents' ineptitude in initiating the process that it takes him three volumes to get himself born. Accounts of scientific research are often presented in a non-Shandean form suggesting that the process was planned in advance to follow a logical and ordered sequence from a body of known knowledge to a target that had been defined at the initiation of the project. A timetable appears to have been set, and landmarks on the way to the final goal established to monitor progress. Some scientific projects—particularly applied science with a definable goal—do follow this path, but many do not, especially problems in basic science whose objective is to find the explanation of a natural phenomenon. Science proceeds from one uncertainty to another, serially validating each sufficiently that the next step can be undertaken.

Gary Saul Morson, professor of Slavic languages at Northwestern University, is a literary commentator and critic, an authority on the great Russian novelists Dostoyevsky and Tolstoy. He has stressed that these authors did not want their characters or themselves restricted in their freedom of action; they desired, rather, that events over time—*Tempics*, as he called it—would determine outcome, and that the end could not be foretold in the beginning. *The Idiot* and several of the other great novels were written as serial pieces for a literary periodical. When writing the first chapters, the authors did not know the ultimate ending. Historic events that were included in the later chapters had not even occurred when the first chapters were written and published. The stories are not neat. An incident

---

[2] The historian and sociologist of science Robert K. Merton has elaborated on the theme of Shandean narration in his popular book on the origins of the phrase, attributed to Newton, "If I have seen farther, it is by standing on the shoulders of giants." R. K. Merton, *On the Shoulders of Giants: A Shandean Postscript* (New York: Harcourt Brace Jovanovitch, 1985).

recounted early in the novel may not figure in the later narrative, and not all events are incorporated into the final outcome. Similarly, in our story, things don't always pull together, even though an ordered reason was the predominant guide. But the story does have a pattern, and I hope it will emerge in this book. Don't expect *War and Peace*—but you may recognize some of the apparent confusion that permeates that novel.

There is a story told by a historian who for years had tried to interest his bright young daughter in his subject: bringing books home for her to read, telling her stories, and encouraging her to watch educational TV shows designed to stimulate the interest of the young in our collective past. Nothing moved her. Then, the family took a trip to Rome and spent a day wandering about the Forum gazing at the enormous ruined temples, markets, and palaces that bestrew this reserve in the center of the modern city. His daughter roamed the site by herself for most of the day and, in the evening—her imagination fired by all the possibilities suggested by the great ruins—asked her father, in wonderment, "What happened?" Her interest in history began on that day.

What happened with the discovery of the hepatitis B virus? My colleagues and I at Fox Chase Cancer Center in Philadelphia had a role in its discovery and application to medical practice, and I propose to tell you about it. I want to offer readers (both scientists and nonscientists, I hope) an account of the events that we took part in, and also to give some idea of how scientists work day to day. The scientist gets up in the morning, goes to the laboratory, the clinic, the field, and then—what transpires? I believe that there is insufficient knowledge in the general community of the methods and the processes that scientists use. There is a growing body of literature in this genre, much of it excellent, that helps to make our goals, possibilities, and motivations—what drives scientists—more transparent to those who are not scientists. Although science, particularly in America, is generally well received and often well supported, there is still a suspicion of its process and the resultant products. Industrial pollution, environmental degradation, nuclear weapons, biological and chemical warfare, and many other products of technology are seen as the baleful outcome of the scientific endeavor. One has only to look at the portrayal of scientists in literature and the movies to see the concerns that are conveyed to the public. Mary Shelley's brilliant story of Victor Frankenstein and the Creature he (she) invented and fabricated is a classical tale often retold in print, on the stage, and in the movies. There is a fear in the public mind of creative arrogance, of efforts to mimic natural forms or even to outdo them. This is especially well illustrated in the movie and novel *Jurassic Park*, the Michael Crichton blockbuster. The molecular biologist who is responsible for the recombinant chemistry not only wants to create dinosaurs from the scraps of DNA obtained from an extinct dinosaur's blood found in the gut of an arthropod preserved for centuries in amber, but he strives to improve them. He wants them to grow more rapidly to provide a quick return on the investment of the venture capitalists, and to move more ponderously to fulfill the preconception the public has of dinosaur demeanor. This results in the fearsome outcomes so vividly told and shown.

I hope that the story presented here, along with the many other accounts of scientific research that are now available, will help to acquaint the reader with the process of scientific research and the motivations and generally amiable character of its practitioners.

The story about to be told has a Shandean character, particularly because, at its outset, we did not know we would discover HBV and apply the findings to practical medical and public health purposes. There are roughly three phases to the story that often overlap in time. During my medical school years and clinical house staff training (1947–55) I became impressed with the great variation among individuals and populations of individuals in their response to disease risks. Some became ill and others did not; some responded to treatment well and others poorly; some died and some lived. What were the reasons for these differences? Luck could account for some, but scientific explanations and, therefore, wholesome interventions should also be possible. This period is covered, more or less, in the first two chapters of the book.

The second phase began about 1956 when my colleagues and I started a systematic search for inherited biochemical and immunologic variation ("polymorphisms") in human populations and sought to explain how this inherited variation—"diversity" is the word that is currently popular—interacted with a sometimes hostile environment. Underlying this program was the notion—in fact, the faith—that in due course we would identify inherited differences in susceptibility and resistance to disease, although at the outset we did not know what the disease would be. This portion of the story is covered in chapters 3 and 4, which also include a digression describing the research on physical biochemistry accomplished during my graduate school period. The third part of the story (chapters 5 to 11) begins in about 1965 when, as a direct consequence of our study of biochemical variation, we discovered the hepatitis B virus and invented the HBV vaccine. We shifted our research and dedicated our energies for the next thirty years to understanding how HBV operates and how this information could be used to prevent and treat the disease. Our research eventually turned back to its conceptual origins—the study of variation—and this is described in chapter 12. Conjectures on the future of research in the field—some not firmly rooted in solid data—are presented in the final chapter.

It would be inaccurate and misleading to give the impression that we had a set goal from day one; we did not. The story line isn't direct, but neither was the research—nor, for that matter, is life in general.

In the years following the identification of HBV, other hepatitis viruses—HAV, HCV, HDV, HEV, HGV—have been identified, and still more are likely to be found. Control of these viruses has also advanced considerably, although, in general, not as far as that of HBV. In the early 1980s, the tragic AIDS epidemic became apparent. HIV and HBV have many features in common. They both can be transmitted in human blood. HIV is a member of a class of viruses that can produce DNA from RNA—they are retroviruses. HBV is also a retrovirus, although in a somewhat different fashion from HIV and other "conventional" retroviruses. The epidemiology and methods of transmission have similarities, and many of the risk groups for HBV are the same as those for HIV. The histories of the two viruses have been intertwined in large part because of these similarities, and their research paths were often parallel. Unfortunately, it has not been possible, so far, to develop a vaccine for HIV, although this may happen in time. Lessons that have been learned from HBV research have been and will continue to be of help in illuminating the complexities of HIV.

Prevention of a disease has great advantages over treatment; a goal of modern medicine is to keep people healthy and functional and allow them to live out their allotted times disease-free and in reasonable comfort. HBV vaccine is the first widely used vaccine to prevent a common cancer. Other viruses cause, in part or in the main, several uncommon and common cancers. Included among these are cancer of the cervix, cancer of the nasopharynx, certain forms of leukemia and lymphoma, and probably others. If the current HBV vaccination campaign against cancer of the liver continues to be as successful as the initial results have indicated, then it will be an inspiration to scientists to seek other vaccines to prevent other common cancers.

Hepatitis is a very important disease and has attracted outstanding investigators. I will refer to many of them during the course of the account, but I have undertaken to describe our role in the search for the hepatitis virus and its consequences and have not attempted to write a history of the entire research program. I hope that I have not slighted any of my colleagues, and I assure the reader that comprehensive reviews of past and present work are available.[3]

---

[3] See, for example, the WHO monograph *IARC Monographs on the Evaluation of Carcinogenic Risks to Humans*, vol. 59, *Hepatitis Viruses* (Lyons: IARC, 1994), and W. Muraskin, *The War against Hepatitis B: A History of the International Task Force on Hepatitis B Immunization* (Philadelphia: University of Pennsylvania Press, 1995).

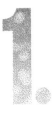

Differences in Response to Disease

A Short Personal History

I WAS BORN in Brooklyn, New York, in 1925, in my parents' apartment in a building my father owned. The family lore was that each time a child was born (there were three of us), an extra room was cleaved from an adjacent apartment to add to ours. Nineteen twenty-five was a splendid birth year. There was relative peace in the world, the only conflict of note in my earliest years being the Gran Chaco War in the remote Andes. The greatest tragedy of the year was the wreck of the Navy dirigible USS *Shenandoah*. The stock market was doing well, and the country enjoyed prosperity as it emerged from the turmoil of World War I. Our middle-class comfort gradually eroded after the market crash of 1929, which greatly hampered my father's career as a lawyer in New York. Twenty-fivers (i.e., people born in 1925) are children of the depression, which has, I believe, instilled in all of us a need for a measure of financial security that we could generate by our own labors.

My grandparents had come to the United States from eastern Europe at the end of the nineteenth century in the great wave of emigration that brought many European Jews to North America and the Western world. I am inexpressibly grateful to the people of that generation, who had the initiative and courage to travel across land and ocean to a new life. Despite their immigrant origins, my father and his two brothers were university educated—my uncle Henry was a professor of mathematics for more than thirty years, at the Universities of Wisconsin and Ohio—and several of my mother's and father's brothers were also university and professionally educated.

I attended a Jewish parochial school in New York—the Yeshiva of Flatbush—for my elementary education, and I have always felt that it gave me an enormous intellectual push at a crucial time in my life. We were at school for nearly eight hours a day. In the morning we were occupied with the curriculum required by the New York State Board of Education. In the afternoons we learned Hebrew, read many of the books of the Hebrew canon in the original language, and, in addition, studied parts of the extensive commentaries on the Torah, the Talmud. This practice introduced us to the fact-based argumentation of these works of critical appreciation, which have a curious kind of reasonable but directed argument that I believe is conducive to modern scientific thought.

I continued my education at New York City public high schools at a time when the intellectual standard and the achievements of their students and graduates were amazing. Far Rockaway High School, from which I graduated, had no fewer than three Nobel Prize winners among its alumni, including the remarkable Richard Feynman[1] and the equally remarkable Burton Richter, who was, for many years, the director of the Stanford Linear Accelerator. It wasn't until I reached Oxford that I encountered an intellectual atmosphere as lofty as the one I enjoyed in high school. It was there that I realized that I would be a scientist. My mathematician uncle, despite his eccentric ways, influenced me, as did a gifted high school chemistry teacher, Lottie Grieff, who encouraged me in my scientific interests. I can also recall a visit from a distant professorial relative who had spent his academic career as a mathematician in Switzerland. I asked him about the theory of relativity and what tensors were (I had read about the latter in a Philo Vance mystery story). He provided an urbane and helpful answer for a teenager. I still remember that on a winter night he did not wear an overcoat, and his only concession to the cold was an elegant pair of leather gloves.

[1] The biography of Feynman (James Gleick, *Genius: The Life and Science of Richard Feynman* [New York: Vintage Books, 1992]) contains a rich description of Far Rocka-

The Second World War was a central experience for our generation. I entered the Navy when I was seventeen and was sent to complete a degree in physics at Union College in upstate New York. I was commissioned as a line officer and served on several small amphibious ships. My last assignment was as captain of one of these. I enjoyed the Navy experience and have always appreciated the lessons I learned: responsibility, which an officer on a small ship has to learn quickly; forward planning with the establishment of contingency options (that is, if plan A doesn't work, plans B and C are already in place); the importance of logistics and infrastructure; and also the strange sense of freedom and closeness to the elements one finds at sea. The sea continued to interest me. After the war I took several trips in the merchant marine, ending my career as a ship's surgeon for the now-defunct Grace Line.

My senior professor and adviser at college, Frank Studer, strongly recommended that I leave physics. He realized sooner than I that I didn't have the specific intellectual skill to be successful in that subject, and at my father's recommendation, in 1947, I entered medical school. I graduated (in 1951) from Columbia University's College of Physicians and Surgeons, at that time one of the best medical schools in the country—and still excellent. Four years of hospital training as intern, resident, and fellow at Bellevue and Presbyterian Hospitals in New York City followed, and then a period at Oxford University, England, where, in 1957, I received a doctoral degree in biochemistry.

In 1957 I returned to the United States. I was a scientific investigator at the National Institutes of Health in Bethesda, Maryland, during a period of rapid physical and intellectual growth when it was, as it is now, a major center of biological and medical research. In 1964 I went to the Institute for Cancer Research (now Fox Chase Cancer Center) in Philadelphia, where I have remained until the present. Perhaps "remained" isn't the appropriate word: during this period I spent several sabbatical years abroad, including a five-year appointment (1989–94) as Master of Balliol College, Oxford University-

---

way, where Richard spent part of his childhood. ("Charmed lives were led by the children of Far Rockaway. . . ." [20])

sity. Nor was I at complete rest during the periods I wasn't actually living abroad. The field trip requirements of my research took me to many parts of the world: West and East Africa, the central Pacific, the Philippines, Australia, South America, China, India, Taiwan, South Korea, Singapore, Hong Kong, and the majority of the countries of Europe.

The Origin of Scientific Ideas

Where do scientific ideas come from? Most scientists can describe an event or a series of events, often casual, that vectored them to a scientific direction that they then followed for many years. Darwin's entry into the world of diversity and evolution came after a series of failures. He was unsuccessful at medical school at Cambridge and, later, recognized that he would not make a good country vicar. Searching for a proper vocation for him, his father arranged for him to serve, unpaid, as the naturalist on the *Beagle* and to provide civilized conversation for its commander, Captain Fitzroy, during the lengthy circumnavigation. His ideas about diversity, evolution, and selection arose gradually as the voyage proceeded, influenced by the writings of his uncle Erasmus Darwin,[2] his reading of Lyell's geological text, which stressed the evolutionary changes brought about by uplift and other geological forces, and his accumulating observations of the great variation in plants and animals living in different parts of the globe. It wasn't until years after his return to England that he fully recognized the broad concept of evolution and selection.

---

[2] Erasmus Darwin had always seemed to be a remote figure until I read a short description of his appearance and activity that firmly placed him in a more human context. In the Harverian Oration of 1986 presented by George Whitfield and entitled "Royal Physicians" (published in the same year by the Royal College of Physicians, London), Dr. Whitfield describes four physicians who did *not* accept the usually coveted position of physician to the royal family. Among these was Erasmus Darwin who "begged to decline without stating his reason, which was that he was hoping to marry Mrs Chandos Pole, a widow, of Radbourne Hall, Derby and there were many other contenders for her hand. Darwin was fifty, grossly overweight, severely

Sir Anthony Epstein, the British virologist, describes how he was motivated to work on viral causation of cancer in humans after, by chance, attending a lecture by Denis Burkitt, a surgeon working in Uganda. Burkitt described a childhood tumor, which now bears his name, Burkitt's lymphoma, that was common in parts of Central Africa, but relatively rare elsewhere. He also reported his epidemiological studies. The prevalence[3] of the tumor was dependent on temperature, elevation, and geography, a finding compatible with the notion that it was caused by a mosquito-transmitted infectious agent. After hearing Burkitt's lecture, Sir Anthony recognized that he should be looking for a virus in the lymphoma. He eventually identified the virus associated with the cancer and was rewarded by having it named after him and his laboratory assistant, Yvette Barr. In this instance, as in many others, there was a prepared mind on which the seed of the idea came to rest and then flower. Epstein had been attempting for years, without success, to identify a virus in the tissues from human cancers. He recognized after Burkitt's talk that his eponymic lymphoma tissue was the right place to look. There are numerous other examples of the circuitous route to scientific discovery.

I believe I know why I started working on inherited and environmental variation in disease susceptibility. By the time I completed the third year of medical school, I had already experienced the great heterogeneity of the population of New York City that our hospital served, and was aware of differences among individuals and among populations of individuals in responses to disease-causing agents. People who were, apparently, equally exposed to a disease-causing agent, such as a bacterium or a virus, could respond very differently. Some would remain healthy, while others sickened; some would respond well to treatment, while others would not. The effect of environment was also obvious: people who lived in favored regions were less likely to be exposed to disease-causing agents than those

---

pock marked and with a marked stammer. He did not wish to add distance to these disadvantages."

[3] In epidemiology, *prevalence* denotes the proportion of a population that is currently infected; it is usually expressed as cases per 1,000 or per 10,000, or may be written as a percentage. *Incidence* denotes the rate of occurrence of new infections per unit of time (e.g., per year).

who lived in other, less salubrious, parts of the world. But the significance of this had not truly registered on my consciousness. Wanderlust was the conduit to my next step. I wanted to spend some time doing medical work in the tropics, and it was there that the questions arose concerning inherited susceptibility to disease and how this reacts with the elements in the environment. Why the tropics? For people of my generation, raised on the movies of the thirties and forties, our major image of the tropics was generated by the Tarzan movies that enraptured my contemporaries and me; we did not at that time recognize these films' blatant racism and condescension to "colonial" people. (Several years in my late teens of after-school employment as a movie theater usher undoubtedly enhanced my attraction to the lures of the silver screen.) This was also a period of romantic reading for me. Joseph Conrad's *Lord Jim* and *Heart of Darkness*, Wallace's *Tropical Nature*, H. M. Tomlinson's *The Sea and the Jungle*, and other stories of hot-climate adventures lured me to experience the jungles and the tropics. Strangely, medical school gave me an opportunity to do this.

Melville at the beginning of *Moby Dick* tells of Ishmael's restlessness and his need to quit the streets of New York, and how his wanderlust drove him to New Bedford and then on to a whaling voyage to the Pacific. I too wanted to quit the winter-gray city and enter the heat and sun of the tropics. With the intercession of our professor of parasitology, Harold Brown, my classmate Jack McGiff and I spent three months at the hospital and public health facilities at an aluminum mine in Suriname, on the northern shoulder of South America. It wasn't until much later that I realized how large an effect this experience had on my thinking and on my subsequent research.

Suriname and Moengo

Suriname, or Dutch Guiana as it was then also known, is now independent, but at the time of our visit in August 1950 it was one of the remnants of the Netherlands' colonial empire in the New World. European influence was minimal. There were a few miles of motor roads along the coast, but the vast forested interior stretching from the Caribbean coast in the north to the dense jungles of Brazil to the south had no roads, no airstrips, and few people. Large portions had not been mapped or explored by Westerners. The indigenous population were South American Indians belonging to various tribes, including the Caribs (whose ancestors had gone on to colonize the Caribbean islands and were among the Indians encountered by Columbus and his followers), Arawaks, Akaways, and other small groups. Europeans came to the country in the sixteen hundreds. In 1654 there was a major influx of Sephardic Jews who came to Suriname from Brazil when the Portuguese overwhelmed the Dutch colony in Recife.

Over the course of the years, other populations were brought into the country to work on the plantations. The first of these were enslaved Africans from the Caribbean and the west coast of Africa. Within a short time of their arrival, they had launched a successful revolutionary campaign against their European masters and by the mid–eighteenth century had signed peace treaties with the Dutch government, which granted them independence in several communities in the interior of the country. Theirs was one of the first slave rebellions in the New World, and one of the most successful. When we were in Suriname, the Dutch crown was still delivering annual reparations to the Djukas (or Bush Negroes), as the self-liberated populations were known. There were five main tribes, descendants of the insurgent Africans, mostly located on rivers south of the escarpment that more or less paralleled the coast fifty kilometers or more south of the Caribbean coast. When the north-south flowing rivers encountered the escarpment, they formed steep and extended rapids. These could be negotiated by *corriales*, large dugout canoes. The Djukas were the only ones capable of bringing boats through the rapids.

Later, indentured workers were brought from what is now Indonesia (then the Netherlands East Indies), and from India. Small numbers of Chinese and other population groups also found their way to Suriname.

The mine and town of Moengo are located about 150 miles upriver from Paramaribo, Suriname's major port and only large city. Moengo began to flourish as an aluminum mine about the time of the First World War, when it became clear that oceangoing ships could navigate the deep but narrow Cottica River and carry up to about seven thousand tons of bauxite ore, the raw material for the production of aluminum. A courageous river pilot, a Surinamer still working on the river when we were there, recognized and pioneered this route. The possibility of transporting huge quantities of ore by ship made the mine's development and expansion economically feasible. By the time of World War II, the mines of Suriname, mostly those of Moengo, were supplying a good part of the bauxite needed for the American war effort.

The Surinaamsche Bauxite Maatschappij (Suriname Bauxite Company), a subsidiary of the Aluminum Company of Canada, ran the mine, controlled the town, and employed essentially all the wage-earning adults in the community. A medical examination was required of all employees before they came to work, and their subsequent health care was supplied at the company-owned hospital. The town was a model of good public health in an area where endemic diseases—malaria, intestinal parasites and bacteria, tuberculosis, yaws, filariasis (the cause of elephantiasis)—and a variety of other serious illnesses prevailed. Clean water and inspected food, inside plumbing or pit latrines, pasteurized milk from its own dairy, and insect control were effectively maintained. Moengo had received routine residual DDT spraying since the 1940s, and malaria, filariasis, and other mosquito-borne diseases were not transmitted within the confines of the community. However, many of the employees brought these infectious diseases with them when they came to the community. Moengo was a heterogeneous society comprising individuals from many parts of the globe with different prior environmental exposures and representing different gene pools. They had congregated in this isolated community and now shared its environment. It was an excellent place to observe differences in response to infectious agents.

There was little or no information on the distribution of infectious disease in Suriname in general and, in particular, on the border between French Guiana and Suriname; we wanted to know about the extent and intensities of these diseases. This information would be useful in the design of public health programs and would add to the general knowledge needed for a basic understanding of how these illnesses were distributed among people living in very different environments. We would also provide medical care for people we encountered during the surveys, most of whom would never have had any previous contact with Western medicine. We did extensive studies on the distribution of infectious agents in Moengo and elsewhere and completed the first surveys of filariasis and one of the earliest surveys of malaria in this region. This involved an exciting trip up the Marowyne River (that is, south) in a *corrial* and through the rapids to the capital of the Paramacanners on Langatabatje Island, as well as many visits to other communities near and distant from Moengo.

The malaria survey showed a striking difference in the prevalence and the character of infection between the villages near Moengo, where medical care was available, and Langatabatje. There were about half as many people infected with *P. falciparum* in the near-Moengo villages as in Langatabatje, which was remote from hospital and public health facilities. In addition, in Langatabatje malaria was classified as highly endemic, while in the near-Moengo villages the rating for this disease was "healthy." This classification is based on the prevalence of palpable, that is, enlarged spleens in the population. Individuals who have been infected with malaria for long periods in certain areas of the tropics develop enlarged spleens, probably as a result of constant exposure to the antigens of the parasites in their tissues. The ratio of palpable spleens to malaria infection was much higher in Langatabatje than in the near-Moengo group.

The officials of the Suriname Bauxite Company were pleased to see these results since they could infer that the presence of their hospital and medical staff had a wholesome influence on the health of the population in their community. This was a possible, but not a necessary, conclusion, as the sampling in both locations was probably too small. Also, there were undoubtedly variables in addition to the effective mosquito control in Moengo that could have accounted for the difference. Despite these uncertainties the malaria survey was a striking field demonstration of the differences in disease response related to environment and geography.

The Filaria Study

The studies on filariasis proved to be the most interesting. *Wuchereria bancrofti*, the causative agent for filariasis in this part of the world, is transmitted via the mosquito (in Suriname mainly *Culex fagitans*) into the bloodstream and internal organs of humans. The male and female filarial worms find each other in the maze of blood and lymphatic vessels, mate, and produce offspring. The infected human host may react to these events with an immune response leading to inflammation in the blood vessels and lymphatic drainage, which may then become blocked. This can result in swelling of the extremities and organs peripheral to the blockage, in some cases causing gross exaggeration of their normal size. Legs, arms, and genital organs of males, particularly the testes, may be involved. A similar disease (caused by a related parasite) is present in the central and south Pacific and during World War II was of considerable concern to servicemen there. It is still one of the major afflictions of the tropical world and one of the diseases selected by the World Health Organization as a special target for intensive attack. In 1998, it was estimated that 120 million people in seventy-three countries were infected with the organism.[4]

A fascinating feature of filariasis is that many of those infected do not become obviously ill but have large numbers of the organisms (the microfilaria form) in their blood. That is, they are "carriers" of the organism although they themselves are not ill. But if they are bitten by a mosquito that, in turn, bites another person, the disease may be transmitted; and some infected people will become sick.

---

[4] Early in 1998, a program to eliminate filariasis was announced by the giant British pharmaceutical firm SmithKline Beecham and the World Health Organization. The firm planned to donate five billion doses of the drug albendazole (worth about half a billion dollars), which can eliminate the parasite from its host. The donated drug and two other effective agents, diethylcarbamazine and ivermectin, which kill the larvae, would also be used. The countries taking part in the program would be responsible for hiring the staff to administer the drugs. It will be a formidable task, since as much as five years of treatment are required to rid the infected person of the agent (*Nature* 279 [1988]: 645).

This pattern of infection is analogous to the carrier status of hepatitis B, which I will discuss in much greater detail later in this story.

Microfilaria emerge at night in South America, but during the day they are hidden in the internal portions of the body. Apparently they respond to activity patterns of their host, and the night emergence favors the transmission of the agent by human-biting mosquitoes that are active after dark. We conducted our survey at night both in the hospital and by visiting the residential areas of the mining community. We collected blood during daylight from the small number of employees who worked the night shift. Since information was available about all the inhabitants of the community and about their comings and goings (essentially only by riverboat), it was possible to have an accurate census and to collect blood specimens from nearly all the employees, many of their family members, and also several peripheral communities that had been established adjacent to the mining town proper.

The results of this study lingered—or, more accurately, became embedded—in my thinking and imagination over the following years. There was a much higher frequency of carriers among the "Creoles" (that is, Surinamers of mixed African and European descent) than among those of Javanese, American Indian, Chinese, or European/American origin. In each of the groups a higher percentage of males and of younger people were measurably infected. Comparison of the Creole and Javanese groups was particularly meaningful, as their numbers were large and most of the people of the two communities lived in company-provided housing, presumably under similar conditions of exposure. The data raised a whole series of questions.

Were the differences in susceptibility to chronic infection—the higher frequency of carriers among the Creoles as compared to the Javanese—a consequence of differences between the two populations in the frequency of susceptibility genes that conferred a greater likelihood of persistent infection? Were the differences in infection a consequence of cultural or environmental differences between the populations? There was an intriguing possibility in the second category. The Javanese cuisine is spicy, very spicy. Often, the only antidotes are vast quantities of beer and time. A Dutch scientist had reported that one or more of these spices contained hetrazan-like compounds, hetrazan being a plant-derived therapeutic that is used as a treatment for filarial infection. Was it possible that the condiments decreased the frequency of carriers? Was the higher frequency of carriers in the males as compared to the females a consequence of "biological" differences between males and females—hormonal differences, for example, or genes on the X or Y chromosomes? Was it due to differences in behavior of the sexes? Were men more likely to be bitten by mosquitoes in the course of their work, or to have more exposure when hunting or fishing?

At this early period of my life as a scientist questions arose that would intrigue and excite me for years to come. How do inheritance, human behavior, and the environment interrelate in the context of disease? At one extreme there is a completely determinist interpretation: genes determine outcome and biology is destiny. At the other stands the view that factors in the environment and human and population behavior influence outcome. But for most diseases all these factors are involved, often in unique and surprising intricate combinations.

This was my first trip to the tropics, my first experience of the region's complex environment, heterogeneous populations, and exaggerated responses. I wrote in my diary:

> Nature operates in a bold and dramatic manner in the tropics. Biological effects are profound and tragic. The manifestations of important variables may often be readily seen and measured, and the rewards to health in terms of prevention or treatment of disease can be great.

Ultimately, the scientific methods that I learned in Suriname had a profound effect on my later research on hepatitis. It was there that I learned to rely on observations in the field; new observations led to new hypotheses that could not have been induced by laboratory-based experiments. The stark interplay of genetic differences and environmental effects was clear in the harsh tropics. But the fieldwork was, in turn, very dependent on laboratory techniques, and hypotheses were confirmed or rejected by experimental testing. Field experience conferred another gift, one that I did not appreciate until much later. In my isolation from telephones, mail, and constant conversation I actually had time to think!

After leaving Suriname in 1950, I didn't return to the tropics for some years. Aside from a small experimental research project on filaria-infected wild rats in my fourth year, I didn't continue research on filariasis after returning to medical school. I had to finish my last year and complete four years of hospital training before returning fully to research. The direction that research would take was influenced by my experiences in Suriname and my observations there of differences in response to infection among different individuals and among populations with different origins, cultures, and behavioral patterns. My clinical experience as a house staff officer and fellow at Bellevue Hospital and at Columbia-Presbyterian Medical Center further reinforced my curiosity about the mechanics of clinical diversity. These adventures informed much of what subsequently happened in my scientific life.

Clinical Experience and Scientific Research

There were many things that I didn't understand during my two years (1951–53) on the house staff at Bellevue Hospital in New York City, but the most mystifying was the outlook of the veterans, doctors who had finished their Bellevue training years ago and returned for nostalgic visits. Dewy-eyed, they told us how wonderful their experiences on the First Division at Bellevue Hospital had been. Vital, rich, joyful—their sentimental recollections were astounding to us. In my view, in those early weeks, it was incredibly hard work—long hours, low pay ($50, later $125, per month, and all found), and equipment that was reminiscent of seventeenth-century Hogarthian institutions.

It wasn't until some years after I left and from the vantage of a more leisurely period of life that I finally realized that the experience of Bellevue was a Dark Passage, a trip like Dante's. Midway in his life Dante found himself in a dark wood, at a bifurcation of a road, and because the right path was lost and gone, he took the left, which led him to a descent into the circles of Hell, through the world and out again under the Southern stars, up Mount Purgatory to the Heavens and beyond, and then to a return to earth. Or like Conrad's hero Marlow, steaming up the Congo River into the heart of darkness, experiencing the fateful rendezvous with Kurtz, and then returning somehow renewed by his experiences of Hell. Dante and Kurtz would have understood the house staff experience at the Bellevue of the time. However, the experience was not all Dantesque. I courted my wife, Jean, at Bellevue, claiming that the food in the house staff restaurant was excellent, and, further, that we had outstanding bread and pastries supplied by the nearby Riker's Island prison.

Our "catchment area" included some of the dreariest areas of the city, and many of our patients were from among the destitute, homeless, often alcoholic men (and a few women) who found a haven in New York not provided in less tolerant communities. As interns, we were given a great deal of responsibility, and we soon learned that if we didn't undertake a task, then it was usually not done at all. The nurses and the other staff were excellent, but there were far too few of them. Tasks that in other hospitals were the responsibility of others—for example, the laboratory studies done at the time of admission, escorting patients to the X-ray department, cross-matching blood for transfusion—were performed by the interns or residents because we knew we had to do them if we wanted to keep our patients alive. Most of the house staff lived in the hospital and were lulled to (much needed) sleep by the cries of the children on the nearby pediatric wards.

Despite all this, our morale was remarkably high. We prided ourselves on the fact that we were never closed to admissions. Other hospitals could declare that all their available beds were occupied, and could refuse to admit even the very ill, but when there were increased demands at Bellevue, extra patient beds were set up in hallways and the ancillary service rooms. It was not uncommon during the winter to have many more patients on a ward than were theoretically allowed by the available beds. We also shared a penchant for enthusiastic recreation. I vaguely remember a party that caught the attention of the New York tabloids: we were celebrating some long-forgotten event in one of the public rooms in the house

staff living quarters. The papers published a vivid account of sup-
posedly excessive drinking and licentious behavior, with a grainy
photograph of the room the morning after, strewn with bottles, cigarette butts, overturned furniture, and difficult-to-identify pieces of
clothing. A feature of their story, to which I can attest, was a description of footprints going up one wall, across the ceiling, and down
the opposite wall. I don't recall how that feat was accomplished.

I loved the excitement of the ambulance assignments; it appealed
to even the least romantic of souls. Called to a "serious case" in that
then mysterious region of lower Manhattan east of First where the
avenues are named with letters (now gentrified as "Alphabet City"),
I could see even before jumping out of the ambulance that it was,
indeed, very serious. Tragically, the victim's head had been crushed
under the wheels of a city bus, and there was no possibility of life. A
crowd was gathered in a semicircle around the scene of the horrible
accident. The police department wreckers were in place, prepared
to lift the bus off its victim; searchlights from fire department emergency vehicles played over the scene. There were warning lights,
sirens, radios: the whole set of props for a medical drama. Caught
up in the spirit of the occasion, I jumped lightly from the rear of the
ambulance, the large greatcoat issued as a symbol of our office
draped loosely over my shoulders (recall General Broulard as
played by Adolphe Menjou in Kubrick's masterpiece, *Paths of
Glory*), the cap emblazoned with "Bellevue Surgeon" set squarely
on my head, my brow cool, eye steady, and jaw set.

"Who's in charge here?" I said, digging up from the littoral of my
memory the vernacular of some long-gone macho hero of a 1940s
movie. (Norman Mailer has wisely said that the memory banks of
our generation, the source of our imagination, are the movies of the
'30s and '40s.) The police officer escorted me to the victim, and the
surrounding crowd began in a low voice the chant, "It's the doctor,
it's the doctor." Encouraged by this totally unexpected public interest (at the hospital we thought of ourselves as low in status and socially invisible), I carefully examined the obviously lifeless body for
vital signs. It was clear that there was nothing that I could do. Light
reflexes gone, no response to stimuli, heartbeat unobtainable, pulse
absent, skin temperature beginning to drop. I even used a mirror to

see whether breath condensed on it, a ritual of little clinical value, but a part of the death mythology of the time. I slowly rose and said, as if to the surrounding crowd, "This man is dead," and to the police, "Could you take him to the morgue?" "He's dead, he's dead, he's dead," echoed the crowd, and I walked slowly back to the cab of the ambulance, departing with lights flashing and horn blowing.

I don't know how you define epiphanies, but I go along with what I think Anthony Burgess had in mind when he used the term: an event, usually a moment in time, that is long remembered and has a symbolic or actual significance, often hard to define, that goes beyond the actual experience. Bellevue had its epiphanies—I think of them as experiential haiku—and I will indulge in the recounting of only one. Many of our patients were homeless, separated from any responsible family connections, and often, sadly, alcoholic. Alex (not his real name) came into the hospital suffering from head injuries incurred in what must have been a very violent street battle. The police were unable to identify the perpetrators—Alex claimed they were "friends"—and turned him over to us for repair. His wounds sutured, he ended up on the medical wards, where he was found to have pneumonia due to a (at that time) rare and difficult-to-treat organism—*Klebsiella*. He was given most of the available antibiotics, but it was touch and go. Finally, after a few weeks of medical care, much of it given by me, and very effective nursing, he showed signs of recovery and was obviously out of mortal danger. I spent a few contemplative minutes with him most days dressing his wounds, which provided us with a little time for casual conversation. He had been a recalcitrant patient, often refusing treatment, probably because of his general despair over his life. But I had insisted that he continue with the program. Now that he was feeling much better, he set about thanking me, which he did in a gracious manner, and then added, "You know, Doc, life is sweet after all."

These moments of high, low, and tragic drama were, however, rare. Most of the seemingly endless time with patients was dedicated to maintaining them and, occasionally, making them whole again. The great variation in susceptibility and response to disease agents was a constant theme of the experience, reinforcing the impressions I'd garnered in Suriname. This was particularly true on the tuberculosis wards. During the period I was at Bellevue, tuberculosis was a very common disease. Really effective antibiotics did not emerge until a few years later, a development that was to lead to an enormous decrease in hospitalized patients, the closing of tuberculosis sanitariums, and, in time, the end of the tuberculosis ward at Bellevue. But it was a very busy place when I was there. It was a truism of clinical folklore, but in fact backed up by research, that certain populations were much more likely than others to become infected with tuberculosis and, if infected, to respond less well to treatment. For example, people of Celtic and Scandinavian origins were thought to be less resistant than the Jews. Although we only rarely saw indigenous American Indians at Bellevue,[5] and I had no direct medical experience with them at this time (I did later, particularly during my field trip to Alaska), it was well known that they were prone to tuberculosis and that Inuits (Eskimos) were even more susceptible. It was obvious that a good part of this increased susceptibility was a result of poverty and all its consequences, but the obvious differences in environment did not preclude inherited differences in disease susceptibility.

Medical Diagnosis and Clinical Research: Comments on Scientific Process

Arriving at a medical diagnosis can be viewed as an example of scientific process. First, a few paragraphs about scientific process in general.

In the *inductive* phase, we first collect data and with them formulate a hypothesis. The notion of "pure induction" is usually associated with the seventeenth-century English essayist and pioneer of scientific method Francis Bacon (1561–1626). It implies that the data are based entirely on the observations without recourse to prior theory or hypothesis. The mind is a tabula rasa, a blank page. However,

---

[5] There were actually many Indians in New York City, including the Iroquois, who were "high-iron" workers (i.e., did the steelwork on skyscrapers) and "sandhogs" (tunnel diggers).

total "blankness" is highly unlikely. "Pure" induction is always modified by some preconception of where the investigation will go. The fact that a decision was made to collect data in a particular place (the beach at Cape Cod, the surface of the moon, the glaciers of Greenland) and within a particular category of nature (plants, mollusks, clouds, quarks, nucleic acids, etc.) indicates the existence of a working hypothesis. In the inductive phase of science there is a prior conception of the direction of the scientific endeavor.

In the *deductive* phase, the hypothesis is stated first, and then experiments are devised and observations made in an attempt to support ("prove") or reject it. Some scientists think that it is never possible to actually prove that a hypothesis is true beyond any doubt.[6] Although multiple studies may support the hypothesis and none rule against it, the very next experiment may provide grounds for its rejection; the uncertainty remains and it is not "proven." On the other hand, it is possible to reject a hypothesis if the predictions generated by the hypothesis are not supported in one or more experiments.

In practice, this is better than it sounds (the very phrase quoted by Mark Twain in describing Wagner's music). If a hypothesis is tested many times and is *not* rejected, and the experimenter is satisfied that subsequent experiments are *unlikely* to reject it, then it can be accepted *as if it were true*. The consequence of this acceptance is that the scientist can proceed to the next step in the program of experimentation regardless of whether the hypothesis is "true" in any absolute sense. One could say that the scientist doesn't deal with truth but is concerned with having sufficient evidence to accept a statement as if it were true, and then moving on with the process.

After the experiment to test the hypothesis is completed, the data are collected and the experimenter decides whether the hypothesis is supported or rejected. Independent of the ultimate fate of the original hypothesis, the data collected to test it can now be used to generate new hypotheses. Usually, one or more of the "new"

---

[6] The contemporary formulation of this idea has come from the writings of the late Sir Karl Popper (1902–94), the Vienna-born British scientist long associated with the London School of Economics.

hypotheses will be a modified restatement of the original, now rejected, hypothesis, enriched by the new information obtained as a consequence of the experiment. One is happy to reject a hypothesis if it is replaced by a more attractive hypothesis, that is, one that has richer and fuller information content than its predecessor. Now this new hypothesis must be retested with a set of data different from that which generated it, and a new experiment must be designed and executed for this purpose.

This pattern may seem obvious, but it is remarkable how often a hypothesis generated by a body of data is said to have been "proven" by it, whereas in fact, this newly generated hypothesis requires a new study design and the resultant body of data to test it. In addition to hypotheses that are restatements or amplifications of the initial hypothesis, the data can also generate hypotheses that are not directly related to the initial hypothesis except by the obvious connection that they originated from it. It is a common experience of scientists that unexpected data are often the most interesting because they generate totally new kinds of ideas. Recognizing this, we began to organize our study design so as to produce unexpected results. This may seem semantically facetious—if you expect something unexpected, can it really be unexpected?—but it works.

New data are produced by each hypothesis tested, and these data in turn lead to additional hypotheses and more data and more hypotheses. The process produces many answers but even more questions. The more you know, the more you know about what you don't know. Einstein put it far more elegantly when he noted that the larger a circle of light becomes, the greater the perimeter of darkness around it. Research is a continuous process with no logically determinable end; it continues to provide more answers and even more questions that broaden the understanding in an, at least theoretically, limitless space. In medical research, answers can be applied to the solution of medical problems, to therapy and prevention, but even a practical outcome does not mean that the investigation is complete.

In clinical diagnosis the first step is inductive. We formulate a hypothesis—that is, a tentative diagnosis—based on the information gained from the presenting complaints, history, and physical findings. We then test the initial hypothesis using additional clinical and laboratory information collected after the first experience with the patient. We generate successive hypotheses and either support or reject them with additional data in a manner similar to the repeated hypothesis formulation and rejection already described. This process continues until we judge that we have sufficient support for a definitive diagnosis. When we do, we assign the patient to this category and institute the appropriate treatment for the disease. I will illustrate this with a hypothetical example.

A middle-aged male, slightly obese, with tobacco stains on his fingers, is wheeled into the emergency ward clutching his chest, breathing heavily, and appearing very apprehensive. The physician, approaching the patient, tacitly induces the hypothesis, that is, makes the tentative differential diagnoses: (1) respiratory disease, probably pneumonia; (2) cardiac disease, probably a coronary artery occlusion. He places his stethoscope on the chest, senses that the patient does not have a fever and, after careful listening, that the respiratory sounds are normal, though rapid. This combination of symptoms and findings rules against primary respiratory disease (although it does not rule it out) but is consistent with coronary artery disease, as is the rapid, somewhat irregular, pulse. The patient is now sufficiently composed to respond to questions and gives a story of a sudden onset of crushing pain in the mid-chest radiating to the arm, which is also consistent with the diagnosis of coronary artery occlusion. A detailed history is now obtained. His father had diabetes and died of coronary artery disease. The history raises another hypothesis/diagnosis of diabetes underlying the coronary artery disease and supports the coronary artery disease. Rapidly, additional independent information is obtained. The X ray taken in the emergency ward, though not of high quality, shows that the lungs are normal in appearance but the heart is enlarged beyond normal limits. Finally, the EKG supports the diagnosis of heart disease.

The doctor repeats the process of formulating hypotheses/diagnoses that are either supported or ruled against by successive collections of data until he or she arrives at a conclusion, *after which action is immediately taken*. A principle that is firmly imbedded in the heart and mind of the physician is that action must follow when a particular hypothesis has withstood the test of rejection a sufficient number of times. The doctor may then prescribe treatment, request further tests to help support the diagnosis or to induce new ones, or he or she may even advise the patient to do nothing. Nevertheless, a decision and a course of action are required before the physician and his patient part.

An interesting feature of this process is that, because of the requirement for action, the earlier decisions are made on the basis of incomplete knowledge. Something must be done soon after the patient enters the emergency ward clutching his chest and requiring relief. The next level of hypothesis making and data collection may add further useful knowledge, but there is always the sense that the decisions are being arrived at without all the information that could conceivably be obtained. Well into the process of firmly establishing the clinical diagnosis, the physician may feel that there is still additional information that would be useful to have, but that would take too long to obtain given the necessity for immediate action of some kind. Medical school, and particularly clinical education, is an exercise in learning how to make decisions with incomplete knowledge.

In 1955 I left the intensive clinical experience of the hospital years and started full-time research. For many years I continued to see patients as an attending on medical services and, laterally, as a consultant. This clinical experience continued to have a profound influence on my research methods, and, in particular, on their application. In the research I did later (of which you will soon learn more) we found a mysterious antibody in the blood of a transfused patient. My clinical colleagues and I recognized that the antibody could be reacting with a hepatitis virus; our experience with disease accelerated what might have been a much longer process of discovery.

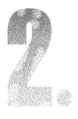

Oxford and the National Institutes of Health: Inherited Variation and Susceptibility to Disease

WHILE COMPLETING my fellowship in internal medicine (1955), I had decided to specialize in research on and treatment of diseases of the joints.[1] My mentors suggested that I undertake a project in physical biochemistry. They assumed that, because of my training in physics and mathematics, this would be a suitable topic for me. Little did they, or I, realize that I had reached the limits of my mathematical capabilities, and this was not an ideal subject for me; my thinking was much more biological than I had imagined it would be. In any case they recommended that I work on hyaluronic acid, a natural biochemical that is a major constituent of the fluid in the joints. Ever the dutiful student, I complied. One of the leading workers in this field was Alexander G. Ogston, a physical biochemist in the Department of Biochemistry at Oxford University. Jean Liebesman and I had married in 1954, and we both wanted to live abroad for a period. The notion of a few years in Oxford was very attractive, and I applied to work in Sandy's lab; after due consideration, he agreed to take me on his team. My original plan was to be a full-time researcher, but Sandy suggested that I work toward the D.Phil.[2] degree at the same time, and I matriculated as a student of

[1] I could trace the reasons for this, but they are not particularly interesting and relate only indirectly to the research that later occupied my life.

[2] Whereas U.S. universities use the Latin form Ph.D. (Philosophiae Doctor), Oxford uses the English version, D.Phil. (Doctor of Philosophy). The story in Oxford is that

Balliol College where Sandy was a fellow; this began a long and rich association with the college. But more of this later.

I spent the next few years working on hyaluronic acid, and some of this research is described in Appendix 2. Hyaluronic acid has become an important molecule in science and medicine for quite different reasons from those that had motivated my project, but after I completed the research for my thesis, I did not return to this field. I had become far more interested in the serum protein polymorphisms that I began to study in the second year of my stay in Oxford. Despite my abandonment of the thesis topic, the years I spent in Oxford were a turning point in my scientific training. Sandy Ogston was a wonderful mentor. He shared a laboratory with his graduate students, and we saw him and he saw us nearly daily. He had a great curiosity about nature, and his research was designed to satisfy this curiosity. Although I later learned the value, and excitement, of practical application, Sandy taught me to follow a problem for its own intrinsic value. He had a very rigorous and quantitative approach to biological science, not common in his day, and he managed to convey this rigor to his students. Sandy molded the scientific personality of his students, including me, and I shall always be grateful to him. I also learned about the vagaries of experimental science, in which the experimenter invents his own world, postulated to be an accurate reflection of the "real" natural world. The experimental model allows inferences to be made about the world it is modeling, but this assumption isn't always correct. Comparing experimental results to the actualities of clinical observation or field studies adds the constraint of reality to the exquisiteness of a carefully designed experiment.

Sadly, Sandy died in 1996, but he had led a long and fulfilling life, and, I believe, one of contentment. I was gratified when his family asked me to speak at the memorial service held, as is the custom for leading members of Oxford University, at the University Church of St. Mary the Virgin. It gave me an opportunity to express my feelings for Sandy and all that he had done for his students.

---

the degree was created for American students, since graduate doctorates were not a popular form of higher degree in the United Kingdom early in the twentieth century.

The intriguing questions of diversity in relation to disease stimulated by my experiences at Bellevue and in the jungle hospital in Suriname continued to occupy my brain and mind. In this chapter, I will discuss some of these principles and how the introduction of a new technical method for the separation of proteins—electrophoresis in gels—allowed our research to vector forward to new discoveries. It also illustrates the reciprocal and mutually dependent relation between science and technology: for new discoveries to be made, new technologies are often required, and new technologies can lead to new discoveries.

Inherited Variation and Susceptibility to Disease

Standing at the foot of a hospital bed, a physician may ask, "Why is the patient sick while I am not? Why in the face of what appears to be equal risk do some people succumb to illness and others remain well?" An obvious response is that some people are luckier than others, and, by chance (the French *par hasard* seems better here), some will be exposed to the cause of the illness and succumb, and others will not. But beyond bad luck, people are different from one another, and some of this difference is related to different biological susceptibilities to disease. An important approach to prevention and treatment in medicine could be to identify differences between individual humans and see how these differences relate to specific disease susceptibilities and to the environment. If we could find them, the most susceptible people could be protected. Further, these differences may reveal details of pathogenesis (that is, how the disease develops in the body) and treatment. Of particular interest are *inherited* differences among individuals and populations that result in differential disease susceptibility, because these can often be detected before the person is exposed to the disease hazard. It was this notion that became the driving force of our research. If we could precisely identify the susceptibility factors before a person became sick, then we might be able to intervene to prevent the illness. The idea of a disease-free life—or, to be more realistic, a life with less disease—might be possible.

Western medicine has traditionally focused on therapy; prevention has, in the past, not received very much recognition. In medical school it was assumed that training in preventive medicine was suitable for public health officers employed by governments, and this was, in the mid–twentieth century, not a high-status professional goal. Studies in disease prevention often include individuals who are exposed to causes of illness but who may or may not become sick. This may be one of the reasons that preventive medicine has never had the allure of other branches of medicine. If everything works well, nothing happens. No one gets sick; no blood, no mad rushes to the emergency room with tubes dangling from arms and legs, masses of equipment covering the patient. It's hard to make a dramatic TV episode out of a no-action scenario.

It was this question of differences that was raised by my experience in Suriname. Why were the Javanese less likely than the people of African descent to become carriers of the microfilaria phase of infection with *Wuchereria bancrofti*? Why, within the different population groups, were some individuals infected and some not? At the time, there were only a few characteristics (ethnicity, age, sex, place of residence) we could examine to account for the differences in the responses. The first problem, then, was to find human biochemical and immunologic characteristics that were practical to study and that might be related to disease. Technical developments beginning in the 1950s facilitated the study of a vast treasury of human variation in the serum proteins that had previously not been readily accessible. I will discuss them—but first, some examples illustrating the early history of the study of inherited biological variability among individuals and among different human populations.

Inherited Biochemical Variation within and between Populations: The Salonika Campaign

In 1916, during World War I, the Allied High Command decided that the terrible stalemate of trench warfare in western Europe, with its enormous slaughter of men and limited gains, could be circumvented by an attack from the south, the "soft underbelly of Europe." Urged on to a large extent by Winston Churchill, at that time the First Lord of the Admiralty in the British cabinet, the military leaders planned a new series of campaigns. The most famous (or infamous) of these was the attack on Gallipoli in Turkey by combined British and imperial forces, which eventually resulted in another stalemate and, later, the withdrawal of the forces.[3]

A campaign was also planned through northern Greece into the Balkans and central Europe. To that end a large military force was assembled in Salonika, the principal city of the Greek province of Macedonia. It included troops from India, Serbia, Poland, Britain, France, and North Africa, as well as local military and civilian personnel. The practice of blood transfusion was still in its infancy, but the principles of typing red blood cells to achieve a satisfactory match between donor and recipient, introduced by Karl Landsteiner and his colleagues in the early 1900s, were in general use in military and civilian medicine. Different people had different antigens, and they could be classified into the well-known blood cell types, A, B, and O.

The physicians in charge of the blood transfusion services in the central laboratories of the Serbian army were Dr. Ludwik Hirszfeld and his physician-wife Hanna. Hirszfeld, Polish by birth, had trained in Heidelberg, Germany, in microbiology and immunology. He had volunteered as a contract physician in the Serbian army at the outset of the war and had taken part in the disastrous retreat of the Serbs following their defeat by the Austrians, through the mountains of Serbia and Albania to the Adriatic Sea at Scutari. Later, he rejoined the Serbian forces in Greece and assumed responsibility for the blood transfusion service.[4]

---

[3] I can recommend the Australian movie *Gallipoli*, which poignantly tells the story of the devastating effect this battle had on the Australian forces; the action is presented from the perspective of a young man killed in a desperate and foolish charge into the massed rifle and machine-gun fire of the Turks. My youngest son was with me when I saw this picture for the first time. Afterward, responding to my shock and sorrow, he said, "C'mon, Dad, it wasn't so bad." I impulsively answered, "Yes, but you're a son and I'm a father."

[4] F. R. Camp, E. A. Fuller, and K. I. Tobias, "Ludwik Hirszfeld—Physician, Scientist, Teacher (1884–1954)," *Military Medicine* 143 (1978): 115–19.

From among the healthy Allied troops in the command as well as locals, blood donors were recruited and tested for their ABO blood groups. (The Rh and other blood group variants now known to be important in preventing transfusion reactions were not discovered until after World War I.) When the data were arranged according to the population group from which the donor was recruited (i.e., French, Serbian, African, Indian, Jewish, etc.), the Hirszfelds found striking differences in the frequency of the genes that determined the ABO antigens.[5] That is, within the populations there were person-to-person differences depending on which of the ABO antigens had been inherited; and, when the populations were compared, there were differences in the frequency of the genes that determined the antigens. The populations could be described and compared to each other based on the gene frequencies.

The blood cell antigens were an example of inherited differences in susceptibility to disease. If an individual had inherited a particular combination of antigens, he or she would be susceptible to transfusion reactions if transfused with blood containing different antigens; if transfused with the same antigens, the person was "protected" against a transfusion reaction. The ABO red blood cell antigens were among the first of the systems of inherited common biochemical traits, called polymorphisms, studied by scientists.

Genetic Polymorphism

During my second year at the Department of Biochemistry in Oxford my research took an unplanned turn, which eventually brought me back to my original interest in inherited variation. There has been a long-standing interest—one could call it a preoccupation—in Darwinian evolution at Oxford, particularly in the Department of Zoology. Oxford was the scene, at the 1860 meeting of the British Association for the Advancement of Science, of the great

---

[5] L. Hirschfeld and H. Hirschfeld, "Serological Differences between the Blood of Different Races: The Results of Researches on the Macedonian Front," *Lancet* 2 (1919): 675–79.

debate between Thomas Henry Huxley, Darwin's colleague and spokesperson (so effective a representative that he was called the "bulldog"), and Samuel Wilberforce, bishop of Oxford. Wilberforce, a strong defender of religious orthodoxy, challenged the notion that humans were descended from lower primates and, in the heat of argument, asked Huxley if he was descended from an ape. Exercising his considerable rhetorical talents, Huxley replied,

> "[A] man has no reason to be ashamed of having an ape for a grandfather. If there were an ancestor whom I should feel shame in recalling, it would be a man, a man of restless and versatile intellect, who, not content with an equivocal success in his own sphere of activity, plunges into scientific questions with which he has no real acquaintance, only to obscure them by an aimless rhetoric, and distract the attention of his hearers from the real point at issue by eloquent digressions, and skilled appeals to religious prejudice."[6]

This devastating reply seems to have defused the argument and advanced the cause of Darwinism.

E. B. Ford, professor of ecological genetics in the Department of Zoology at Oxford, developed the concept of a genetic polymorphism. His definition, which is still useful, is as follows: "the occurrence together in the same habitat of two or more discontinuous forms of a species in such proportions that the rarest of them cannot be maintained merely by recurrent mutation."[7] Admittedly, this is a turgid and information-dense statement, but some examples will help the reader to unravel its meaning.

Ford and his father were lepidopterists; they studied moths and butterflies mostly in the English countryside. One of the best and earliest examples of polymorphism came from the the the Fords', and other zoologists', study of these insects. In 1846 the first example of a mutant form of the moth *Biston betularia* was reported in southern England. It was black. The common form (*typica*) of *B. betularia* in this region of England in the mid–nineteenth century had a mottled

---

[6] Quoted in Alexander B. Adams, *Eternal Quest: The Story of the Great Naturalists* (New York: G. P. Putnam's Sons, 1969), 389.

[7] E. B. Ford, *Genetics for Medical Students*, 4th ed. (London: Methuen, 1956), 101.

gray-and-white wing coloration. This pattern provided effective camouflage protection for the insects. It was very difficult to see them when they rested on the lichen-covered oaks and other hardwoods characteristic of their habitat. The black form (*carbonaria*), determined by a single dominant allele, was presumably a consequence of a chance mutation from the common mottled form.[8] They were rare, because specific mutations from one to another form of a gene are rare, and predatory birds would much more readily eat the black forms that did mutate. The frequency of the black gene in the population would be maintained only by recurrent mutation; it would therefore be at a very low level—one in a few thousand. Beginning in the mid–nineteenth century and continuing into the twentieth, the melanotic (black) forms became more and more common in many areas of central and southern England until in some regions they nearly completely replaced the previously common mottled forms, which now became the rare variety. What had happened to cause this remarkable change in the appearance of a common species of moth?

The Industrial Revolution came early to Britain and was accompanied by the widespread use of coal in the industrial areas of England. Vast amounts of pollution resulted, and in this region (the "Black Country") many of the lichens covering the trees were killed. The tree trunks assumed a more uniform and dark appearance, and the melanotic black *Betularia* was now better protected against predation than the mottled form. Many examples of color changes of this nature (known as industrial melanism) are known from Britain, Europe, and elsewhere.[9]

Another well-known example of a polymorphism is sickle-cell hemoglobin disease (sickle-cell disease), often discussed in elementary

---

[8] Different forms of a gene, called "alleles" (singular, "allele"), may be present in different individuals at the same location ("locus") on a chromosome. Individuals may have one or another depending on the form they have inherited from their parents. New alleles are sometimes generated by mutation at a particular locus and may then be passed on to subsequent offspring.

[9] Industrial melanism in *B. betularia* has been, for many years, presented as a classical example of polymorphism and natural selection. Recently, doubt has been cast on

biology courses. Hemoglobin is a protein in red blood cells that is essential for the transport of oxygen. Most people have normal hemoglobin A in double dose (genotype Hb^A/Hb^A)—that is, they received a Hb^A gene from both their mother and their father. In some regions of the world, including many parts of Africa, southern Europe, and portions of Asia, an alternative allele, Hb^S, which produces sickle-cell hemoglobin, may be common. Individuals with two of these genes (homozygous Hb^S/Hb^S) are likely to develop sickle-cell hemoglobin disease, which can decrease survival because of the limited ability of sickle hemoglobin to transport oxygen. It also produces detrimental effects by clogging blood vessels. However, young people who are heterozygous, Hb^A/Hb^S, are protected against death from falciparum malaria, a common infection in regions where sickle hemoglobin is common. Each time a person who is homozygous for Hb^S fails to contribute his or her genes to the next generation, because of death or less-than-average fertility, two Hb^S genes are removed from the population. In the absence of any selective factors in favor of the Hb^S gene, the prevalence of Hb^S would drop to a level that could be maintained only by recurrent mutation, that is, at a very small number. But because of the advantage conferred on the heterozygote—that is, sparing of death from malaria—he or she is able to contribute more genes to the next generation than bearers of the other genotypes, and the Hb^S gene is maintained at relatively high levels in the population. Anthony C. Allison, of whom I will have more to say later, was one of the pioneers in establishing the relation between the sickle-cell hemoglobin polymorphism and protection against falciparum malaria. This was based on a series of field trips in East Africa, some of them undertaken under the auspices of the Oxford University Exploration Club, a student club that encouraged scientific and other travel among its members.

The original concept of polymorphism implied that there are survival benefits conferred by some combinations of alleles that other combinations do not provide, and that there is heterozygote advantage. However, it has been difficult to demonstrate advantage for

---

the observational and experimental data that support the original interpretations. (See *Nature* 396 [1998]: 35.)

many polymorphic traits. It is possible that polymorphisms are se-
lectively neutral and occur as a consequence of chance. In many in-
stances the selective advantage of a single polymorphic system
taken by itself may be too small to detect. But if a given polymorphism is considered along with other polymorphic traits and with
environmental factors with which they could interact, selective advantage may be detected.

Independent of the question of selection, the polymorphic systems provided an excellent mechanism for studying biochemical
and immunologic variation among individuals and among human
populations. In the mid-1950s when our work began, the red blood
cell antigens were the most studied human polymorphisms. In addition to the ABO and Rh systems, which were used clinically to ensure compatible blood transfusions, there were many other red
blood cell antigen polymorphisms—for example, Lewis, Duffy, Kell,
Lutheran, Kidd, and Diego—often named after the patients whose
blood was used for reagents to detect the antigens. These were used
in studies of polymorphisms and by physical anthropologists to
characterize and compare populations according to the distribution
of these genes.

The technique used was to collect blood specimens from a sample
of the population in question and determine the frequency of the
antigens in the various systems. From this the frequency of the
genes that were known to control the antigens could be inferred.
The population could then be described by the frequency of these
genes and compared to other populations with which they might
have affinities. There was already a considerable literature on the
population distributions of the red cell antigens, often with conjectures on differences in disease susceptibility associated with different alleles. The notion was that the frequencies of the alternative
alleles would differ from population to population, depending on
the disease and the evolutionary history of the populations, both
remote and recent.

In addition to the red cell polymorphic systems, several other
human polymorphisms were known. Some were rather bizarre; for
example, the ability to taste the chemical phenylthiocarbamide,
tongue twisting, and the presence of an odoriferous material in the

urine after ingestion of asparagus. For the most part the chemical characteristics of these traits were not understood, and one can imagine that their esoteric nature did not convince people that they would be of survival value.

A major step forward occurred in 1955 when Oliver Smithies (who had also been a student at Oxford University of my doctoral program mentor Sandy Ogston) introduced the technique of electrophoresis in gels. Oliver is a remarkable scientist. In addition to his considerable contributions to theoretical biology, he was a great tinkerer. He had vacated the laboratory that I subsequently used when I came to the Department of Biochemistry in 1955, and had left behind the remains of a wonderful constant-temperature bath of unique design that he had built, as well as other more sophisticated pieces of equipment. In addition he was an outstanding small plane aviator and holds several records for long-distance (including transatlantic) flights.

The gel method of electrophoresis has made a great difference in the advance of modern biological research: it is the basis of many of the methods used to separate nucleic acid segments that are essential in molecular biology analyses. Prior to the availability of Oliver's gel methods, scientists accomplished electrophoretic separation by placing a solution of proteins (for example, blood serum) on a wetted paper or cellulose acetate strip. The strip was then placed in an electric field, and the proteins would migrate to one pole or the other dependent on their electric charges, distributing themselves along the strip. Seven or eight different blood proteins could be identified by this method. The gel method allowed the separation of proteins and other chemicals as a function not only of their charge differences but also of their mass and shape, since the proteins had to sieve through the pores of the gel. Twenty or so proteins could be identified initially, and many more with improvement in the gel methods. Using this method, Smithies found a polymorphism of the serum protein haptoglobins (that bind hemoglobin), and there were indications that other polymorphic serum proteins could be identified on the gels.

I did most of these early studies in collaboration with Anthony C. Allison. Tony was a junior faculty member of the Department of

Biochemistry when I arrived in Oxford to start my graduate research. We became good friends. His second son was born about the same time as our first child, his wife was an American, and he and I were both twenty-fivers (i.e., born in 1925). But our backgrounds were quite different. I was brought up American and urban. Tony was the son of a Kenya planter and was brought up in the highlands of then-colonial Kenya. He obtained his medical school education in South Africa and a doctorate from Oxford. Tony was involved in population genetics and was fired up by the concept of polymorphism. As I have already related, he led several expeditions to East Africa that provided some of the earliest findings on the relation between sickle-cell polymorphism and falciparum malaria. He encouraged me to read E. B. Ford, J.B.S. Haldane, R. A. Fisher, Sewell Wright, and others who had pioneered the field of human population genetics and polymorphisms. It began to dawn on me that the study of human polymorphisms would provide a conceptual framework for the investigation of inherited human variation and its connections with disease and survival, and that the gel method of electrophoresis could be a main technique for identifying the variation.

The style of the research was very appealing. It would require travel, working with populations outside of Western culture, and the prospect of active searching in the fashion of the explorer-scientists of previous centuries. I would dredge up the geographic knowledge I had amassed in my youthful hobby of stamp collecting in the selection of locations for field trips. Our grand plan was to track the distribution of the polymorphic traits in populations living under very different environmental conditions, where the health risks would vary greatly. We expected that different disease risks would have generated different selection pressures, and that the frequency of the genes determining the polymorphisms would vary.[10] Also, we would be more likely to find previously undiscovered associations between disease and polymorphisms. But we had no idea

[10] Academic scientists have to find a disciplinary bin in which to categorize their research. I called my research section at the National Institutes of Health "Geographic Medicine and Genetics." Slightly awkward, but it made it easier to get authorization for field trip travel expenses.

what disease associations we might find. As we learned, scientific discovery has interesting and unexpected turns and outcomes.

During the following years I undertook many field trips to collect biological specimens for the study of polymorphisms. It was a form of inductive science—that is, collecting data within a general conceptual framework, but without specific hypotheses; the hypotheses would be formulated after the data had been collected. These quests were the main thrust of my research for the next decade or more, and I will describe several of these projects. It was during the course of our study of human polymorphisms that we, unexpectedly, discovered the hepatitis B virus.

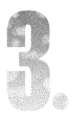

Polymorphisms and Geography: Disease, Genetics, and Evolutionary Biology

IN THE 1950s there were only a handful of scientists interested in polymorphisms, a subject that seemed far too esoteric and removed from medical applications. Polymorphisms were used in forensic studies, to establish paternity, to a limited extent in blood banking, and by anthropologists who compared populations based on the makeup of their gene pools. There was a particular advantage in the application to anthropology. Biochemical traits were, mostly, not visible and did not carry the burden of bias that skin color, eye color, or other obvious traits sometimes did. Polymorphisms have become of much greater importance as the Human Genome Project has developed and more and more genes have been found to be polymorphic. Detecting polymorphisms is much easier at the DNA than at the protein/amino acid level. They can be used to identify individuals who would have a higher probability of responding to drugs, who would develop side effects to drugs or be more susceptible to disease, and to pinpoint other characteristics that would be of great value in disease treatment and prevention. All this was to be in the future; now, we were starting a systematic survey of populations to determine the distribution of

Portions of this chapter have been adapted from B. S. Blumberg, *The Publications of Baruch S. Blumberg Series on Twentieth Century Biology* (Singapore: World Scientific Publishing Company, 1999).

known polymorphisms and to search for new polymorphic bio-chemical traits.

By late 1956, while I was still in Oxford, techniques became avail-able for the study of inherited biochemical polymorphisms, tech-niques that could be used to identity differences among individuals affecting their susceptibility to disease. The general question had been formulated by my experiences in Suriname, in particular the striking differences in the frequency of filaria infection between the Indonesians and people of African origin who were living under apparently similar levels of exposure in the company-built facilities in Moengo. The concept had been hammered home by my experi-ences at Bellevue, particularly on the tuberculosis wards, as I have already described. A good part of the differences in susceptibility to tuberculosis was a consequence of poverty and poor living condi-tions, but a central premise of our approach was that environmental and genetic factors always interacted and that the obvious differ-ences in environment could interact with inherited differences in disease susceptibility.

However, our strategy did not call for a direct attempt to find gene-disease relations. That was too risky. At the level of knowledge that existed in the 1950s, there was insufficient data on inherited biochemical variation, and even fewer clues on how this variation might be associated with disease. Years ago, the Yale undergraduate newspaper published a sophomoric parody of the New York *Daily News* that included fake advertisements. One was for a fictitious school of dance; the text read (if I remember correctly), "If you can walk, you can dance. We will teach you to walk." We decided we were going to learn to walk—that is, we were going to try to find new kinds of inherited variation and determine the distribution of the genes in different normal populations living at extremes of envi-ronment. Later, we would learn to dance, that is, find the associa-tions between the polymorphic variation and disease. Smithies's starch gel technique was going to be the technique that we would use to find genetic patterns in serum protein variation.

The concepts we planned to use were derived from human evolu-tionary population biology; they were based on established con-cepts, along with some derived inferences.

1. *Disease is an important selective factor in human populations, that is, disease affects human evolution.*

2. *Different populations living in different environmental conditions will be subject to different disease hazards.*

3. *There are geographic differences in environment and in disease distribution.*

4. *The differences in disease may be absolute (i.e., frostbite rare in Florida, more likely in Greenland, malaria more likely in West Africa than in Sweden, etc.) or quantitative (i.e., tuberculosis is more common in Inuits in Alaska than in people in Palo Alto, California, but it does occur in the latter at lower frequency).*

5. *The genetic pools of populations living in different geographical locations will differ from one another. These differences will, at least in part, be a consequence of the differences in the selective effects of diseases. These differences may be large when there are extreme differences in disease patterns.*

6. *As a consequence of the emigration of many populations over the course of human history, populations of different geographic origins often live in the same country and share the same environment. These populations may have somewhat different gene pools even though they will share many genes in common. These gene pools are a consequence of the selective factors peculiar to the populations' original homeland that have operated over the generations prior to their emigration to the new region. The differences in the distribution of the ABO blood types in different populations in Salonika during World War I have already been described.*

7. *The gene pools of emigrant populations from different geographic origins may become more similar over time as a result of both intermarriage and the operation of similar selective forces (i.e., the diseases prevalent in the new geographic region) on the previously separated populations. For example, Africans in sub-Saharan Africa have a high frequency of the sickle-cell trait that is due, partly, to the selective effects of falciparum malaria. Americans of African descent have a lower sickle-cell frequency than Africans living in Africa, but a higher frequency than Americans of European origin with whom they now share a similar environment. This lower frequency is a consequence of* *both gene admixture, resulting from intermarriages between members of the two populations, and the lower selective effects of falciparum malaria in North America.*[1]

Edward O. Wilson, in his fascinating scientific autobiography,[2] describes how in the 1960s and 1970s he and his colleagues developed similar concepts linking ecology, evolution, geographic differences, and genetics. His data were in large part derived from his intensive studies of ants living in the same and in geographically separated locations. His work was extended to the behavior of other species and led to the formulation of his ideas on sociobiology—that is, the effect of genes on individual and social behavior—which subsequently became controversial when the concepts were extrapolated to the behaviors of humans. It was another example of the argument that arises in various forms throughout the history of applied genetics. Is a trait inherited and therefore unchangeable, or is it due to environment and therefore subject to change by human intervention? In a real sense, this is a nonquestion since most, if not all, biological phenomena are a consequence of both genetics and environment, and it is often very difficult to disentangle their complex interaction. Furthermore, the effects of genes can be changed. A person who has diabetes that is at least in part inherited may be treated, and the effects of the genes mitigated. Or if a person has a genetic susceptibility to diabetes, avoidance of the appropriate environmental factors may delay or even abort the development of symptoms. Disease may be "caused" by behavior, as in the case of sexually transmitted diseases such as hepatitis B or AIDS, and it may be

---

[1] Indigenous malaria is now rare in the United States. However, before the successful antimalarial campaign conducted during and after World War II (based to a large extent on the use of DDT), falciparum malaria was very common in the southeastern United States, affecting hundreds of thousands of people annually. Although imported malaria is not uncommon, cases that originate in the United States are rare. An endemic occurred in the rice-growing regions of the Central Valley of California, where the malaria was imported in infected immigrants from India and spread by local mosquitoes.

[2] E. O. Wilson, *Naturalist* (New York: Warner Books, 1994).

much harder to change self-destructive behaviors than to intervene to change the effects of genes.

So we had the hypothesis—inherited biochemical variation is related to disease susceptibility; we had the technique—electrophoresis in starch gel; we knew where the populations were that differed from each other in disease prevalence—essentially everywhere; we had the motivation and the urge for questing. All we needed was the money to fund the research, and that came pretty readily.

The Basques of Spain

We started our survey on the distribution of polymorphisms with studies on populations in Great Britain, primarily around Oxford, to obtain data from a European population that could then be compared to others. I had been invited to present a scientific paper in Spain and was given money to do so; this provided the opportunity to obtain blood specimens from another population. Early in the morning of September 15, 1956, we piled into my VW bug, drove to Dover, and ferried to France for a leisurely drive with several pleasant meals at *centres gastronomiques* on our way south; there ensued a short stay in Madrid for the conference, which was wonderfully disorganized but extremely pleasant, and then a journey to San Sebastian on the northern coast of Spain in Guipuzco, one of the provinces of the Basque region.

The Basques live in several provinces bridging the western portion of the border between France and Spain. They encompass the Bas Pyrenees, beautiful green and wooded low mountains, with many hectares of rich pasture for grazing of sheep, a traditional Basque skill. These people were willing to live the lonely life of a pastoralist, and many have migrated to the United States to herd sheep in the vast open spaces of Nevada and elsewhere in the West. In 1957, in Franco's Spain, there was among the Basques a strong element of opposition to the highly centralized government. However, life appeared peaceful.

It was because of their unusual language that we were prompted to study the Basques. Nearly all European languages are members of the Indo-European language family, which includes Greek, Latin, Albanian, the Romance languages, English, German, and Dutch, among others. Basque has no fundamental affinities with these (although many French and Spanish loan words have been introduced), and it is not clear with which languages it is associated. The linguistic scholarship in the 1950s had it that Basque had affinities with several languages of the Caucasus region and possibly with Berber languages spoken in the High Atlas Mountains of North Africa. The view when we were doing our studies was that the Basques were an ancient autochthonous European population which over the centuries had intermixed with other populations migrating from the east and south. In any case they were considered to be culturally and genetically different from other Europeans. Since we were attempting to study populations that were deemed to be different and may, over the centuries, have had different environmental experiences, the Basques were a suitable study population. Additionally, it would not be a very expensive project since we were already going to Spain and had the promise of collaboration with Spanish colleagues, who would arrange for collections and provide expert knowledge.

Genetic differences were already known. There was a significantly higher prevalence of the Rh-negative blood group gene in Basque populations. We could surmise that this led to an increased number of Rh-incompatible babies in this population compared to populations with a lower frequency of Rh-negative. If an Rh-negative mother conceived an Rh-positive child, then the mother could develop antibodies against Rh, and this could lead to massive destruction of blood cells and death of the fetus. There would be a resultant decrease in fertility in the Rh-negative mother, unless, to compensate for the loss, there was an increased number of pregnancies. E. B. Ford,[3] the pioneer of polymorphism studies to whom I have already referred, reasoned that there must be an advantage to the Rh-negative genes in the population to compensate for this loss, but there was none obvious. Ever since the population distributions of the red blood cell antigens were appreciated, there had been stud-

[3] E. B. Ford, *Genetic Polymorphism* (London: Faber and Faber, 1965).

ies to determine whether they were related to disease susceptibility. For example, one of the first associations reported was an increased susceptibility to death from bronchopneumonia in group A as compared to group O babies; but it was not confirmed in later studies, possibly because of the widespread use of antibiotics. Here is an early example of the blunting of genetic susceptibility by the exercise of medical intervention. In the 1950s it was found that group A was more common among those who developed cancer of the stomach, and numerous other associations have been reported since then. However, the blood group disease susceptibilities did not have much of an impact on the practice of medicine. The notions of risk and probability were difficult to convey then as they are now, although the advance in the knowledge of the human genome that has occurred in the last half decade is likely to have a big effect. I will come back to this in a later chapter.

The loss of the Rh-positive child of an Rh-negative mother could be averted by replacement transfusion of the baby at birth. Immunization of the mother early in pregnancy led to the near abolition of the Rh incompatibility problem in well-served medical communities. There were also several other blood groups that differed in the Basques. Our studies confirmed the low frequency of B and Fy^a that had been reported earlier by others. We also found that the distribution of the genes of the serum haptoglobin[4] polymorphism did not differ from that of other European populations. These findings were of interest to anthropologists and historians but did not add greatly to our knowledge of inherited susceptibility to disease. The collected results were another brick in the edifice of the data on gene distributions but far from the "breakthrough" that marks success in science. However, it fit into our plans of continuing to increase the knowledge of gene distributions.

---

[4] The haptoglobins bind hemoglobin and recycle it. Hemoglobin is released into the blood when, in the normal life cycle of red cells, they die, break up, and release their constituents into the blood. In certain diseases, such as malaria, when red cells break down much more readily than in uninfected individuals, large amounts of haptoglobin may be required to retain the hemoglobin.

Nigeria

To obtain information on populations with a different environmental experience, we had to go farther afield than a neighboring European country. Africa was the ideal location for such a study. My colleague at Oxford, Tony Allison, had spent his youth and early adulthood in Kenya and South Africa and knew the continent very well. With his knowledge and connections we began to organize a field trip to Africa.[5] But, first, money would be needed for the trip. In 1957, U.S. government funding for basic research was just beginning the acceleration that characterized its growth in the decades to come. I applied to the National Institutes of Health under the provisions of a little-known method of funding. When a scientist had a good idea that needed only a few thousand dollars for its execution, application could be made in the form of a simple letter to the appropriate official. If the proposal was sound and looked as if it had promise, the complex review that was essential for other grants could be bypassed and the money approved very rapidly. I wrote to Bethesda, explaining our project, and was shortly informed that the money would be made available. Flights were booked and I was on my way to my first of many trips to Mother Africa.

Airplane trips in the 1950s seemed more adventuresome than they do now, and West African Airways Corporation's flight WT 921 did not disappoint. The plane was an "Argonaut," a Canadian version of the DC-6, and although our trip was not as eventful as that of the original followers of Jason, it had its moments. Shortly after our departure from London, I noticed that one of the propellers was stopped. Soon, the captain got on the speaker to tell us that a "drop of pressure" had been indicated on the oil gauge and we would have to return to London, which we did after discharging large amounts of gasoline over the English Channel. We were soon on our way again in another aircraft, bound for Rome. We didn't quite make it. On our first attempt to land we were warned off be-

---

[5] In the event, Tony wasn't able to go on the field trip, but I managed pretty well on my own.

cause of a thunderstorm and the presence of several military jets that had lost contact with the tower. We headed for Nice for an emergency landing. I had the impression that the captain had not previously had the opportunity to land there, for our first attempt, which was aborted early in the process, appeared to be directed at the well-lighted main street of the beautiful resort city. After reconsideration we set down at the authorized strip at the airport.

We were up early the next morning and had a pep talk from the captain telling us all how well we were doing. There were many British schoolchildren on board returning to Nigeria to rejoin their families, mostly British Colonial Service staff, for their school vacations. They were typical British kids, well-behaved and unflustered by the hectic trip. The next day we made it to Rome and then to Libya, our first stop in Africa. We departed at dusk out over the Sahara, and, from the relatively low altitude at which prop planes flew, we could see lights on the oil rigs, trucks driving through the night, and the campfires of lonely caravans. Another severe thunderstorm marked our landing at Kano in northern Nigeria, and the sudden equatorial dawn greeted our arrival at the final stop in Lagos, then the capital of the country.

Nigeria was still a British colony preparing for independence, which would come in 1960. In contrast to Kenya, Uganda, and South Africa, Nigeria had few white settlers, probably in part because of the inhospitable climate and the prevalence of disease. West Africa was known as "The White Man's Grave" primarily because of the great mortality caused by malaria. I exercised the health discipline that was deemed so necessary for travelers in the tropics in the days before big international hotels, rapid and frequent jet travel, and the ill-conceived notion that modern medicine can save an incautious visitor from any disease he or she might contract. That meant constant protection against mosquitoes, eating only cooked food—no fresh fruits unless you could peel them, no salads—and drinking boiled and filtered water, or, where appropriate, bottled beer. Staying healthy in the tropics still requires a certain amount of preparation and effort.

I was greeted at the airport by Professor B.G.T. Elmes, chair of the Department of Pathology at the University of Ibadan, and his wife, who were to be my hosts. Ibadan was the major city of West Nigeria and of the Yoruba, the major ethnic group in the region. The Yoruba have a very rich culture that has spread to other parts of the world, imported amid the horrors of the slave trade. Many Yoruba words are incorporated into the languages of African origin of the southern United States and the circum-Caribbean area. These include Gullah, still spoken on the Sea Islands of South Carolina and Georgia (where, several years later, I took part in further health and prevention studies), the Talkee-Talkee of Suriname, and the special dialects of Jamaica, Trinidad, and elsewhere. I spent most of my time in Africa in the company of Yoruba, both while I was in West Nigeria, their homeland, and during my subsequent trip north. They were great company; Yoruba parties were happy and uninhibited events.

There was at least one cultural gift that I acquired from my Yoruba friends. I would occasionally see groups of people marching along the road or assembled in a public place, all dressed similarly, playing drums and musical instruments, talking animatedly. I was told that they were members of an age group, people who aggregated as a social unit because they were born in more or less the same year. It seemed like a great idea, going through life with people with whom you shared a great deal if only because you and they were born at the same time. When I returned to the United States, I formed such a loose social confederation, and I still number among my closest friends 1925ers, people born, as I was, in 1925; many made it through to 2000, and we celebrated our seventy-fifth year together at a four-day millennium party.

The medical school at the University of Ibadan had been in existence for only a few years at the time of my arrival. The academic staff were mostly white Europeans, primarily British, with a few African physicians and academics. They were preparing to Africanize the staff as Independence Day grew nearer. I attended several of the faculty meetings and was impressed with the high morale and the desire of the academic leadership to develop not only the best medical school in Africa but one that would rank with the best medical schools in the world.

I spent the next few weeks collecting blood specimens from several nearby Yoruba villages. Then, on 11 August 1957, we started on a trip to the north to collect bloods from one of the indigenous populations, the pastoral Fulani. The university had provided a monster of a long-wheelbase Land Rover,[6] an automobile I came to admire greatly. Along with the vehicle came an experienced driver who had served in the Nigeria Regiment of the West African Frontier Force in the Burma campaign during the Second World War. A medical student, Oyo Oyefesu, was asked to accompany me during the trip, which he did. Shortly before we were to depart, the servant who was responsible for my quarters at the medical school implored me to take him as well. He had never been in the north and had family he wished to see; he volunteered to serve as my valet during the trip. I had little use for a valet, my wardrobe being very limited, but I knew he could be helpful in the biological collections. At some point on our way north his cousin, who also wanted to visit family, joined him and became a member of the party. The number of people who showed up to ride in the Land Rover each morning seemed to increase as we went along until we had a sizable group taking part in the expedition. I enjoyed the company.

The Fulani swept into sub-Saharan Africa in the early nineteenth century and, in a series of holy wars, established a reformist Muslim empire. Many have become urban dwellers and intermixed with the predominant Hausa culture. A portion have remained pastoral and nomadic, and their economy is based on the cattle they graze over large areas of their former domains. I was seeking the latter group. Some intelligence work was required for us to find out where they were, and a fair amount of trekking over the countryside in the effort to locate their semipermanent villages. We would hang out at marketplaces looking for Fulani who had come to trade; we frequented bars, pubs, and restaurants to learn the whereabouts of their villages. The first collection was near Kaduna, and a second near the District Office in Pankshin. The Fulani were a pretty independent bunch, and it often took a great deal of *palaver*[7] to convince

---

[6] A gift from the Rockefeller Foundation to the university to be used for scientific and medical fieldwork.

[7] A West African pidgin word derived from the Portuguese, meaning a parley, conference, or discussion, with much talk.

them that they should donate blood for our studies. When I arrived at Pankshin, I was greeted by the local medical officer, who recommended that I not attempt a collection. The head tax on cattle had recently been raised, and the Fulani herdsmen were in a belligerent mood. There was a history of violence in the region. I was told that a district officer (a British colonial official) had been killed there some years ago, and I thought it wise to delay the collections, which were obtained some weeks later by the doctor and his colleagues.

During this period my party and I stayed at the West African Trypanosomiasis Research Station in Vom, near Jos, the major city of the plateau area of northern Nigeria. There I met Robert Desowitz, an American parasitologist, who later in his career was the Raffles Professor at the University of Singapore and later still was on the faculty of the University of Hawaii. Bob and I went upland game shooting (I didn't hit anything); as fellow New Yorkers, we had a great deal to discuss. When we had dinner years later in Oahu, we reminisced about my stay in Vom. He told me that the staff at the research station thought that I was mad to attempt to collect blood from the Fulani. I was surprised that they considered it so risky, and annoyed that no one had bothered to tell me of the potential hazard. Bob is a colorful scientist, one of the few Americans to have served in the British Colonial Service, who has written several popular books about tropical medicine with such intriguing titles as *New Guinea Tapeworms and Jewish Grandmothers*[8] and *Who Gave Pinta to the Santa Maria?*.[9] The grandmother reference in the first title concerns infection with *Diphylibothrium latum*, a parasite of freshwater fish that is rendered noninfectious by cooking; grandmothers, preparing gefilte fish,[10] would sample the uncooked fish and become infected. (*Pinta*, in the second title, is a nonvenereal form of syphilis.)

Bob was also a noted big game hunter, in a period when that sport was more accepted than it is today. At lunch one day he showed me a letter from an official requesting that he join several other hunters

---

[8] R. S. Desowitz, *New Guinea Tapeworms and Jewish Grandmothers: Tales of Parasites and People* (New York: Norton, 1987).

[9] Robert S. Desowitz, *Who Gave Pinta to the Santa Maria* (New York: Norton, 1997).

[10] Seasoned chopped fish.

to kill a lion that had been terrorizing villagers and their cattle. Parasitologists lead a rich life.

What was gained from this trip? We published several papers, among them a description of the distribution of the red blood cell groups in the Yoruba and the Fulani and studies on several serum protein polymorphisms, including the hemoglobin-binding haptoglobin proteins, the iron-binding transferrin proteins, and the *Gm* gamma globulin groups. These results have been used in subsequent studies of the population genetics and anthropology of these regions. We also formulated hypotheses related to disease susceptibility. For example, we found that haptoglobin appeared to be absent in many of the Nigerian samples. Since haptoglobin binds free hemoglobin, we conjectured that in Africa, where breakdown of red cells owing to malarial infection is common, the absence of haptoglobin would be disadvantageous; a great deal of iron would be lost through renal excretion, and the African diet is low in iron to replace the loss. This had a resonance in our later studies on the relation of ferritin, the iron-binding protein present in cells and blood, to the presence of hepatitis B virus in the carrier state and the subsequent development of liver cancer. We also suggested that there might be some compensatory selective advantage related to the unusual distribution of haptoglobin genes in the African populations that would compensate for this loss of iron. It was a good try at finding a disease association, but we did not have very substantial data. The scientific world passed it by without notice.

The field trips and polymorphism studies were primarily inductive investigations. We had a broad hypothesis: that the genes determining polymorphic alleles would have different distributions in populations living in different environments and at risk for different diseases. But we did not have a more specific hypothesis. Our primary intent was to make observations in the field and in the laboratory in the expectation that we would observe relationships with health and disease that would generate hypotheses that could be tested more directly in subsequent studies. In testing a hypothesis, the scientist seeks to be economical—that is, to collect just that amount of data, in the laboratory, the clinic, and the field, required to provide a rigorous test. However, there is an advantage to collecting additional data in the same venue—both geographic and intellectual—to permit the testing of additional hypotheses that may or may not be related to the original studies. In many of our field trips we studied organisms in addition to humans to determine whether the polymorphisms found in humans were also present in other animals. This is analogous, on the phenotype[11] level, to the current practice in the Human Genome Project of simultaneously determining the genomes of other species in addition to those of humans. The parallel body of data is extraordinarily useful for the identification of genes and their functions, findings that can then be translated into useful information about humans.

In Nigeria, we found a previously undetected polymorphism in the alpha-lactalbumin milk whey proteins of cattle (*Bos bovis*), which has been of interest in subsequent studies in other laboratories. We also studied the hemoglobin polymorphism in cattle in collaboration with A. D. Bangham, then at the Institute of Animal Physiology in Babraham, near Cambridge, England. Most northern European cattle (and most American cattle) have a single hemoglobin designated A. But Jersey cattle have a high frequency of hemoglobin B that is also found, although in lower frequency, in Brown Swiss, Charolais, Limousine, and a few other breeds of cattle in central and southern France. On the basis of archaeological and other evidence it had been suggested that Jersey cattle originated in the Indus Valley civilization in India and Pakistan and migrated or were brought by nomadic herdsman through Asia and Africa to Europe. We found that the Nigerian White Fulani breed, humped animals similar to the Zebu cattle of India, also had a high frequency of hemoglobin B. We suggested that this might be construed as collateral evidence of the similarities of the Jersey, Indian, and African cattle. We also attempted to correlate the hemoglobin distribution with protection against trypanosomiasis, a common and damaging disease of African cattle. Two breeds of Nigerian cattle, the N'Dama and Muturu ("Coast shorthorn") are resistant to trypanosomiasis and do not

---

[11] That is, by looking at the product of the genes (the proteins), rather than the nucleic acid sequences (the genes themselves), which can be identified now but could not be in the 1950s.

have hemoglobin B, while the Fulani cattle are not resistant and do have hemoglobin B. It was a rather feeble association that did not, to my knowledge, engender very much interest. Altogether, no breakthroughs, but a solid body of data added to the reservoir of knowledge of inherited diversity.

I undertook the Spanish and African studies while I was still a graduate student at Oxford University completing my thesis on hyaluronic acid. Sandy Ogston not only allowed me to make these diversions from my thesis topic; he encouraged me. He knew when to allow students to follow their peculiar interests.

The National Institutes of Health (1957–64)

My wife, Jean, and I had been living pretty much on a student's income, not too big a problem for depression babies, but now the situation changed. My next move was to a real job, with a salary, taxes, and our first home. In 1957, I joined the Division of Clinical Research at the National Institute of Arthritis and Metabolic Diseases (NIAMD) of the National Institutes of Health in Bethesda, Maryland. In addition to my research activities I saw patients at the Clinical Center of the NIH, primarily those with arthritic complaints. There was an expectation that I would continue with my laboratory studies in hyaluronic acid, but they were less exciting than polymorphisms and field trips. Trials of various steroid hormones for the treatment of rheumatoid arthritis and other diseases were a primary mission of the clinical research group; these were important but, to me, unrewarding scientifically and clinically. Taking advantage of the freedom that was encouraged at NIH, I continued my field and laboratory studies in polymorphisms. Over the next few years we undertook field trips to Greece, the Pacific Islands, among Native Americans, and in Mexico and South America. However, I don't think that my work was understood or appreciated. It was difficult to classify it by scientific discipline. It was thought to be epidemiology, which at that time was not considered a very rigorous science. The director of research of NIAMD at the time was DeWitt ("Hans") Stetten, a brilliant scientist who had made significant contributions to the biochemistry of intermediate metabolism. My sense was that he had respect only for a reductionist laboratory approach to biological science—that is, that all biology could be explained in terms of chemistry or physics—and population studies involving whole peoples were considered to be inexact. Years later, when I had been awarded the Nobel Prize, Hans called to congratulate me. He said, candidly, that at NIAMD he had not really understood what I was doing, but that I had been funded just in case I knew something they didn't. This came as a surprise to me, as I had always thought that I was one of the favored scientists in the division. So much for my powers of self-evaluation.

Where did these studies on polymorphisms lead us? As the rest of this book will reveal, they resulted in the discovery of the hepatitis B virus (HBV). But there were many deviations on the road to this fortunate outcome, and I am going to try to lead you through them. In part, I do this to illustrate the Shandean process of science, and, I hope, to demonstrate that this apparently aimless course does have an internal rationale.

We had studied European populations and populations living in the tropics. Where could we go to study an even more extreme difference in environment and history? It was obvious: the Arctic. We had a little money left over from the grant I had received for the Nigeria trip, and I wrote to the National Institutes of Health to ask them whether it could be used for another expedition. By return mail they agreed, and I started planning for a boreal adventure.

The American Arctic

Can you join Air Force medical research group proceeding to Barrow, Wainwright, Point Hope, Alaska, departing Thursday. Rendezvous Ladd Air Force Base 0900 2 July 1958. Immediate reply requested.

A concisely worded military telegram came unexpectedly to my newly established laboratory at the National Institutes of Health. For several months I had been trying to arrange the complex logistics for a trip to Alaska to collect biological specimens from Native Americans—Inuits (Eskimos) and Indians—to continue the polymorphism study. I wanted to do my studies in conjunction with other health surveys so that the people would not have to be bled unnecessarily, and combining objectives would also decrease the cost.

I had not been making much progress with the several authorities in Alaska whom I had contacted, and the offer from the Air Force was a great help. Within a few days of receipt of the telegram, I was at Ladd Air Force Base near Fairbanks, where I was issued arctic clothing and survival equipment, including a parachute that, happily, was never needed. I joined a group of scientists from the University of Oregon as well as Air Force personnel who were studying the role of nutrition in the development of heart disease in Inuits. There was a great deal of interest in the 1950s, as there is now, in the relation of diet to heart disease. It was thought that Inuits ate a very high fat diet, although there was not very much evidence that they actually did. At that time the military, with its large budgets, was able to fund basic medical research. The armed forces had excellent transportation and other facilities and the funds to support scientific groups in the field. Anthony Allison also took part in this trip, but he and I visited different communities in an effort to obtain as wide a distribution of populations as possible.

Early the next morning the members of the group (eighteen of us, including the crew of the aircraft) and four tons of equipment and supplies were loaded up the ramp and into the hold of a commodious twin-boomed twin-engined Air Force freighter. It was neither pressurized nor extravagantly heated. We walked around to keep warm and heaped on the survival clothing we had been issued. As we headed north from Fairbanks, we gained altitude to clear the Brooks Range, and at fifteen thousand feet the air began to get noticeably thin. A few of the group used the oxygen provided, but as soon as we had cleared Mount Doonerak, the highest peak in the range, we started descending to the landing strip at Barrow on the edge of the Arctic Ocean. We managed to land just before a heavy fog came in from the sea, from which the ice pack had just cleared. After the fog closed in, we were unable to leave for three days. Several planes that came in after us had a very difficult time landing. They attempted multiple approaches to the strip before they dared to put the wheels down on the ground, or, in some cases, turned back to land at a safer field.

We spent the time profitably at the Naval Research Laboratory at Barrow, a highly successful laboratory that had supported a large and productive research effort for more than twenty years. I went on several field trips along with the permafrost research group in a "Weasel," an amphibious vehicle adapted for use on the tundra. Late one afternoon while we were out on the tundra in the Weasel, we suddenly heard the engines of our aircraft starting up; apparently the weather had cleared sufficiently to encourage the pilot to try a landing at Wainwright, the locale for our planned field study. We raced back to the station, grabbed our personal equipment, and were soon in the belly of the aircraft and on our way.

The landing strip closest to Wainwright was adjacent to a DEW (Distant Early Warning) Line radar station, one of a large chain of defenses across the sub-Arctic that had been established during the Cold War to warn of possible Soviet airborne incursions. The strip was several miles across the tundra from Wainwright. I was sent ahead to tell the village leaders we had arrived and to ask for their help in transporting our huge mound of equipment to the village. It was bright and sunny as I set off; the rich bird life, the masses of wildflowers, and clouds of insects enjoying the midday warmth gave a tremendous vitality to the scene. The wonderfully clear air and the bright sun just beginning to sink toward the horizon (below which it would not drop for another month) were exhilarating. The path led around the lagoon that separates Wainwright from the mainland, and as I approached the village, I could see the radio tower and church steeple. The ominous sound of dogs barking reminded me of how nasty sled huskies could be. This was before the era of snowmobiles, and dogs were still used for transportation. There were several teams of them lying on the ground, fortunately all chained to stakes. Inuits keep their dogs under strict restraint and do not trust even to rope or leather to secure them, knowing that they can gnaw through anything but chain or wire.

Wainwright consisted of a series of weathered frame houses built just back from the Arctic Ocean shore and dating from the time of the whalers, who had set up trading stations around which the Inuit community eventually congregated. There were 219 adults and children in the village at the time of our visit. As part of the general survey, I examined 111 of them and, during the next week, collected blood specimens, which were to be used to determine the distribution of the polymorphic traits. Red blood cell antigens deteriorate with time, so I was anxious to start the specialized blood testing. The Air Force medical party would not be airlifted out for more than a week, possibly too late to preserve the antigens. Unexpected help arrived late one afternoon when a single-engine Cessna landed on the beach edge. There was no airstrip at Wainwright, but at low tide a small plane could—carefully—land and take off successfully. The pilot of the plane, a man in his early seventies, had run low on gas and had come down in the hope of refueling. He was a former World War I fighter pilot who had been a bush pilot in Alaska for twenty years or more. My preference among pilots in Alaska was always for older people; the rationale was that natural selection would, in the course of time, have eliminated all but the most able of fliers.

He agreed to take me back to Barrow if I could hurry. I quickly assembled my kit and the biological specimens I had collected, and stuffed them into the back of the plane. We climbed to about two hundred feet, leveled off, and started the flight to Barrow, keeping to the coast to maintain navigational contact with landmarks. Bush pilots did not seem to favor high altitudes, feeling that if you could see the ground, you knew where you were. We circled the site where Will Rogers and Wiley Post had died when, in 1935, their small plane crashed during an attempt to circumnavigate the globe—a lonely last place on earth for these two. Then on to Barrow where I spent the night separating the red blood cells from the fluid portion of the blood to help in the preservation of the samples during shipment. Soon they were on their way to Boston, where my colleague Dr. Fred Allen, Jr., would test them.

For the next few weeks Tony Allison and I traveled from one community to the next collecting blood from Inuits and from the Kuchin group of the Athabascan (Na-dene) Indians who lived in the interior regions. Our studies of the distribution of the Athabascan Indians' and the Inuits' blood groups were the most extensive that had been available up to that time, and they still are a resource used to compare populations to one another on the basis of their genetic (or, more correctly, phenotypic) composition. The Canadian anthropologist E. J. Szathmary, in a 1984 paper,[12] used our data in an extensive comparison of American Indians and Inuits from Alaska, Canada, and elsewhere. This analysis supported the hypothesis that Inuits and Indians had different remote origins in Asia.

The distribution of the genes that determine the various types of haptoglobins differed greatly in the Inuits from what we had observed in the European and African populations we had previously studied.[13] A rough analysis of the data suggested that there was a north-south cline (gradient of change), and that the Hp^2 gene was more common in northern than in southern populations. From this we could infer that there were selective factors in the north that favored the Hp^2 gene—presumably something to do with the differences in climate—but we had no clue as to what that might be. This gives some idea of the barrenness of the data and the difficulties of finding selective factors in the pre–Human Genome Project days. Today, the genes could be identified, and there could be an indication as to function, relatedness to homologous genes in other animals, and real clues as to the nature of the selective factors.

The distribution of haptoglobins in the small hamlet of Anaktuvuk Pass, situated in a relatively inaccessible location in the Brooks Range in northern Alaska, was very different from that of the other Inuit populations of Alaska. The haptoglobin type 1-1 phenotype (i.e., homozygous for the Hp^1 gene) was more than twice as high as in the other Inuit populations. This was probably due to the "Founder effect." The village had been established in 1951, only seven years before our visit. It consisted essentially of five families who had previously belonged to several nomadic and seminomadic groups elsewhere in the interior and on the coast. Although hapto-

---

[12] E. J. Szathmary, "Peopling of North America: Clues from Genetic Studies," *Acta Anthropogenet* 8 (1984): 79–109.

[13] B. S. Blumberg, A. C. Allison, and B. Garry, "The Haptoglobins and Hemoglobins of Alaskan Eskimos and Indians," *Annals of Human Genetics* 23 (1959): 349–56.

globin 1-1 type was, in general, relatively rare in the Inuit population, one of the Anaktuvuk elders, presumably by chance, was this
type. Any selective effects that might have decreased the prevalence
of the haptoglobin 1-1 phenotype had not had time to operate in the
population. Again, we could not define the disease association that
might be operating on the haptoglobins, but it was a field day for
all kinds of wild conjectures, with which I will not burden you.

Phenylthiocarbamide (PTC) is a compound with a characteristic
thiourea grouping (that is, it includes nitrogen, carbon, and sulfur).
It has the unusual characteristic that some people taste it as bitter
and others do not. This dimorphism was discovered when a chem-
ist, searching for a sugar substitute, synthesized the compound. As
is the practice of organic chemists, he tasted it and found that it was
bitter. A colleague in the laboratory was not able to taste it, and subsequent family studies showed that the ability to taste the substance
was an inherited trait. The chemical grouping associated with the
taste dimorphism is also present in several antithyroid and goitero-
genic substances, and there is a significantly higher frequency of
nontasters among patients with certain kinds of goiter than among
controls.[14] We determined the frequency of the trait in the Alaskan
Inuits—the first time this had been done—but the numbers were too
small to determine any disease associations.

We collected sera from various Arctic mammals to see whether
they contained proteins equivalent to the inherited serum proteins
found in the humans. These included the Alaska fur seal (*Callorhinus
ursinus*), ground squirrel (*Citellus parryii* barrowensis), and marmot
(*Marmota caligata* broweri). Their molecular size and weight could
be used as a basis of comparison, as could certain functions they
had in common. For example, we studied the serum haptoglobins
that were identified by their ability to bind hemoglobin, presumably
a physiologic function, hemoglobin, albumin, and other serum proteins. We found that the mammals had proteins that were equivalent

---

[14] A goiter is an enlargement of the thyroid gland associated with iodine depriva-
tion. It is common in mountainous and other regions where dietary iodine is scarce.
In 1960 I went to Ecuador to arrange a field trip to study the relation between the
taste test and endemic goiter. There was a major change in the government shortly
after my visit, and I was unable to reestablish my contacts and complete the research.

to the human polymorphism proteins and in most cases differed only marginally from the human protein. From this we could infer that the genes were very similar. These studies, which were among the first to compare the inherited protein phenotypes of humans and other animals, raised an interesting series of questions. How long did it take, in evolutionary time, for the genes and the proteins they determined to change, from one species to the next? How did biochemicals evolve over the years in response to the needs of different species of animals and to their changing environments? This work provided an early insight into the similarities in the genomes of humans and other species. There is a remarkable conservation of genes—that is, the same or very similar genes are found in organisms ranging from the most simple to the most complex. Nature seems to prefer recycling old genes to creating totally new ones.

While in Wainwright I also did a study of the prevalence of several forms of arthritis in the population. As part of the general medical survey, X rays were taken of most of the inhabitants. These were scored for the presence of osteoarthritis, a disease usually associated with advancing years. Oddly enough, comparable published studies were not available from other American populations, but we were able to obtain unpublished data on the distribution of osteoarthritis in a sample of the general U.S. population. There was a lower frequency of osteoarthritis in the Inuits, and this finding was supported by similar studies that were done many years later. It is still not clear why this difference exists.

What had we accomplished in the field studies in Africa, the Arctic, and elsewhere? Primarily, we had added to the store of knowledge on the distribution of a large number of polymorphic traits in humans and in other animals. At the time, before it was possible to determine polymorphisms of the DNA itself, we had laboriously studied the phenotypes, the serum proteins and cell antigens that were the products of the genes. Today, using the much simpler DNA polymorphism procedures, scientists can study thousands of polymorphisms. However, the problem of population distribution remains the same. We must determine the distribution of traits in non-hospitalized populations, as a control, before we can determine whether there is a higher frequency of an allele in a disease population, or whether individuals with a particular allele are at greater risk of incurring a disease. Fieldwork is still necessary.

We had also made a few feeble attempts at determining whether there were disease associations. Our conjectures about the role of the hemoglobin variant in the African cattle in relation to trypanoso-miasis, about the north-south cline of the haptoglobin gene, and several others even less noteworthy were examples of this. But our main goal was inductive: adding to the "stamp collection" of data on polymorphism distribution. This required a certain amount of patience—waiting for the right set of observations that could lead to an important hypothesis about disease association and an understanding of the biological mechanisms that underlay it. The greater the number of keenly observed population distributions, the greater the probability of discovering a suitable hypothesis. We pressed on.

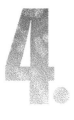

We Discover a New Polymorphism: The Ag System

So FAR, SO GOOD. We were beginning to gain a place among the folks in the polymorphism world—that is, the scientists who were looking for inherited variation in blood and other readily testable human traits. But we were mostly studying traits that had been discovered by others. True, we had found some new ones— for example, the alpha-lactalbumin in cow's milk, a polymorphism of the prealbumin proteins in nonhuman primates that bind thyroxin (whose description I have spared you)—but what we really needed was a polymorphism that had not previously been detected in humans. New polymorphic systems enhanced our chances of finding the disease associations that we lusted after. Having one's own trait conferred a measure of status in the circumscribed world of the polymorphism hunters. It meant that others would send biological specimens for study; it ensured a place at scientific meetings and greatly increased the rate of publication. New discoveries and new ideas require new techniques, and such a technique was soon forthcoming. The discovery not only identified very interesting disease associations but, by the miracle of chance, led us directly to the hepatitis B virus.

In 1960 Tony Allison, my colleague from Oxford who had previously joined me for the fieldwork in Spain and Alaska, came to spend the summer working in my laboratory at the National Institutes of Health. Tony recommended that we try a new method for finding inherited differences in serum proteins. First, an explanation of the rationale of the technique. The work that we had done, and research by other polymorphism mavens, had made it patently clear that there were many polymorphisms of serum proteins, and that the distribution of the alleles (the different forms of a gene that can occupy a particular locus on the chromosome) varied greatly from population to population. The frequency of the alleles of many of them were such that if a patient received several blood transfusions, he or she would have a high likelihood of receiving a protein variant that had not been inherited. If the protein were antigenic (that is, capable of causing an immune response), then the transfused individual might develop an antibody against this slightly foreign protein. For example, consider the hemoglobin-binding serum haptoglobins, the first of the polymorpisms described by Smithies. The distribution of the different phenotypes in a U.S. or northern European population was as follows: 10 percent of people would have inherited the haptoglobin-1 protein, 35 percent the haptoglobin-2 protein, and 55 percent would have both.

Consider patients who have only the haptoglobin-1 protein. They constitute 10 percent of the population and have a probability of 90 percent of receiving a transfusion from a person who has inherited the haptoglobin-2 protein. That is, they would be receiving a foreign protein even if it differed only slightly from the haptoglobin-1 that they inherited. If the haptoglobin-1 patient received as few as five transfusions, the probability of "foreign" exposure would be extremely high. Similarly, if a patient has inherited only haptoglobin-2, the probability of receiving the foreign haptoglobin-1 in a single transfusion would be 65 percent and in five transfusions would be extremely high. Heterozygotes would have both proteins and would not regard either as foreign. So, for 45 percent of the patient population who received as few as five transfusions, the likelihood of receiving a foreign haptoglobin protein was very high. This is analogous to the well-known problem of red blood cell transfusion: a clinical reaction will occur if the transfused blood contains a different red cell antigen from that present in the patient receiving the blood.

There were similar distributions for other protein polymorphisms.[1] and we could infer that either one of the known polymorphisms or something new—a polymorphism that had not yet been detected—might be revealed by the study of sera from transfused patients. The simple hypothesis was that some patients who had received multiple transfusions would develop an antibody against an inherited antigen variant present in the blood of the donor that they themselves had not inherited or, possibly, acquired. This antibody could then be used as a reagent to detect the antigen variant in the blood of the donor, or in the blood of another person in the population who had inherited the same protein antigen variant. The technique we devised was simple: we would obtain samples of blood from patients who had received multiple transfusions and then test them against a panel of sera from other people. We planned to use bloods from different populations in the panel, for we knew that the frequency of the alleles for polymorphisms varied greatly from population to population. We wanted to maximize the probability of finding a new polymorphism.

The technique we used was double diffusion in agar gel, using the Ouchterlony[2] method recently introduced by its eponymic inventor. Holes are cut in a thin sheet of agar cast on a glass plate. The serum from the transfused person is placed in a central well, and sera from the test panel are placed in adjacent wells around the center. Antibodies (that is, special proteins, gamma globulins, produced by the immune cells of the transfused patient that are specific for the foreign protein with which he or she has been transfused) diffuse into the agar. The proteins from the other sera in the peripheral wells also diffuse into the agar, and if the protein specific to the antibody is present, the combined proteins come out of solution and form a line of precipitation in the gel. The precipitation arc can be visualized, or the precipitated proteins can be stained for later study.

---

[1] For example, the gamma globulin groups (Gm), the proteins that migrate just behind albumin in gel electrophoresis (Gc), transferin, the iron-binding protein (Tf).

[2] O. Ouchterlony was a professor at the University of Gothenburg in western Sweden, a noted authority on immunology.

It takes time for the diffusion to occur, and we routinely set the experiment up during the day and put the vessels containing the plates in a bin overnight. We returned the next morning, opened the bin, and, with a keen sense of excitement, examined the plates to see whether any of the precipitin arcs we had hypothesized were present.

Nothing happened with the first few samples of blood from transfused patients, but we persisted. On about the thirteenth try Tony and I entered the laboratory in the morning, opened the bin, quickly looked at the plates, and saw that, adjacent to most of the peripheral wells, there were gracefully curved arcs of precipitated protein. The magic of prediction from a hypothesis had been realized![3] An idea in our minds had, with that visualization, become a reality. We designated the "new" precipitin the "Ag protein," a nonspecific name that vaguely recalled that we had been seeking an antigen. Now, we had to determine whether the variation was inherited and, if so, what protein was involved. We surveyed many normal populations and populations of patients to learn something about the distribution of the Ag protein.

From these first experiments we could formulate several hypotheses to guide the studies to follow. First, the presence or absence of

---

[3] Hypothesis formulation is an exercise in the use of the imagination to explain data and to make predictions. Shakespeare's insight on the magic of poetry evokes this feeling of reality emerging from fantasy in this passage from *A Midsummer's Night Dream*, act 5, scene 1:

> The poet's eye, in a fine frenzy rolling,
> Doth glance from heaven to earth, from earth to heaven;
> And as imagination bodies forth
> The forms of things unknown, the poet's pen
> Turns them to shape, and gives to airy nothing
> A local habitation and a name.

The similarities between artistic and scientific creativity are fascinating. When, in 1982, Jean completed her course at the Pennsylvania Academy of the Fine Arts, I spoke at the graduation about the scientific process and the work of the artist. An example I cited was the difficulty of knowing when a piece of creative art is completed and when an experiment is completed. Both in science and in art, the process is continuous and never finished.

the mysterious protein was a discontinuous trait; that is, you could classify most individuals as positive or negative, and only a small percentage were indeterminate. Second, there was a big difference in the prevalence of reactors in different populations; for example, about 60 percent of the U.S. populations were reactors, but 98 percent of the sera from Pacific Islanders reacted. We then looked for Ag in the serum from several families—mostly mothers, fathers, and their children—and with these data tested a genetic model. In the matings in which both parents were positive and those in which one parent was positive and the other negative, there were both positive and negative offspring. But in the families in which both parents were negative, *all* the children were negative. In addition, in families with a single positive parent either the mother or the father could have the protein. This was consistent with a Mendelian model of autosomal recessive inheritance. This means that there was a gene locus on an autosome—not the X or Y sex chromosomes—that controlled the presence or absence of the trait. If the person had the gene we designated Ag^A in either single or double dose (i.e., had inherited the gene from either parent or from both), then he or she was a positive reactor. People who had inherited the gene we designated Ag without a superscript (implying that we did not know its product) from both parents were negative reactors. That is, Ag^A was dominant to the recessive Ag gene. Later, we tested and retested this model with additional families, and the results were consistent with the autosomal dominant genetic hypothesis.

We had found a polymorphism, but we didn't know exactly what the protein was except that it was an antigen and we could describe its migration in an electric field in electrophoresis experiments. What should we do next? There are many variations of scientific process, and in this case we decided to take a very direct approach. I assembled the immunodiffusion and electrophoresis experiments, visited colleagues at the National Institutes of Health, and asked them the simple question, "What do you think this is?" I obtained a variety of answers, most of them related in some way to the research interests of the scientist I questioned. One of my last visits was to Dr. Howard Goodman, later the director of the immunology program at the World Health Organization in Geneva. He was working on serum lipoproteins (serum proteins that are combined with fats) and, after a few thoughtful moments, proclaimed that it must be a lipoprotein. He was right. We tested his hypothesis and quickly discovered that the precipitin band stained with fat-specific dye, and that it had electrophoretic and other characteristics identifying it as a low-density lipoprotein.

Thereupon followed an intense period of research that continued until about 1968. The initial antiserum had been found in the blood of a patient (Mr. C. deB.) with an unusual form of refractory anemia, never satisfactorily diagnosed, who required frequent transfusions. Mr. C. deB. was a charming and gracious Hungarian emigrant of noble descent, an active member of the Knights of Malta. The whole project depended on Mr. C. deB. Although he lived in the Midwest, he returned to the NIH frequently for medical evaluation and treatment. But he also took a keen interest in our project, and he became a good friend of the members of our scientific team. He supplied us generously with his blood to continue our assays, and even when he couldn't come east, he made certain that we had an adequate amount. Even though our research did not have any immediate prospects of helping Mr. C. deB., he was quite happy to assist us. He told me that if he had in his control something that could be of value to others, he had an obligation to supply it. A very positive civic attitude.

You could say that the population of the world was divided into two groups of people: those whose blood reacted with C. deB.'s blood and those whose blood did not. We subsequently found antisera in other transfused patients that reacted with different specificities of the low-density lipoprotein. A group of investigators, mostly in Europe, became involved in the project, and the genetics began to emerge. There appeared to be a closely linked series of genes that determined complex antigenic specificities. We found a disease association: there was a higher frequency of Ag in patients with diabetes than in controls. From this we inferred that Ag^1 was a susceptibility allele for this disease. In 1976 Kare Berg from the University of Oslo, Norway, working with Curtis Hames, from Claxton, Georgia (who later helped us with the Australia antigen work), showed that one of the Ag phenotypes, Ag(x), is associated with increased serum cholesterol and triglyceride levels. That means that the allele is a susceptibility gene for increased risk of cardiovascular and probably other diseases as well.

At a meeting at the World Health Organization in Geneva in 1970 research workers in the field tried to establish a standard for the antisera reagents to compare the results in different laboratories. But this proved very difficult to do for a variety of reasons, one of which was the variation in specificities we found in testing different antisera. There was also a dispute about the genetic model and the nomenclature to be used, which proved very difficult to resolve.

A few years later, a way forward was illuminated by Kare Berg's development of standardized antisera; he immunized experimental animals to identify specific human serum lipoproteins. The animal antisera defined another human gene locus (Lp), not linked to the Ag locus, that also related to the low-density lipoproteins. Individuals with the Lp(a) phenotype have an increased risk of developing cardiovascular disease. The research on inherited lipoprotein variation eventually led, in the 1980s, to the discovery of susceptibility alleles for human cardiovascular disease. Further research in several other laboratories resulted in the identification of other inherited variations in lipoproteins that are related to the individual's risk of developing Alzheimer's disease. Another example of how the vector of research often leads down a circuitous track whose end is difficult, if not impossible, to discern at its start.

Things were going pretty well in our program to study polymorphisms, discover new ones, and find their connection to disease. But then there was a sudden change that, as you have now come to expect, was unexpected. The wind switched, and we were sailing off in a new and challenging direction.

The Discovery of Australia Antigen

IN 1964, after spending more than seven happy years at the National Institutes of Health, I moved to Philadelphia, Pennsylvania, to continue my research at the Institute for Cancer Research (later named Fox Chase Cancer Center),[1] where I have remained for more than thirty-five years. Timothy Talbot, the director of FCCC, had asked me to come as the associate director for clinical research.

Why did I leave the NIH? It was, and is, a great institution, with an enormous number of talented scientists and excellent resources. I was going to a much smaller place (but with an excellent scientific reputation) to start a new activity from scratch away from the protected environment of a huge government laboratory: no Mama, no Papa, no Uncle Sam, as the street urchins used to cry in our former colonies. My main problem at the NIH, and it took me some time to realize this, was fitting what I wanted to do into the discipline-determined rigidity of the constituent institutes.[2] My research ranged over several disciplines. In addition to the laboratory work, I had to understand the anthropology of the populations we were studying and do field work and epidemiology. I was interested in

---

[1] Fox Chase is a residential community in Philadelphia in the western end of what is known as "The Great Northeast" of the city.

[2] The several institutes that made up the NIH were mostly named for and dedicated to particular disease categories, e.g., cancer, infectious diseases, arthritis, metabolic diseases, heart, neurological diseases, etc.

how the environment and the host interacted to affect the risk of disease, and I didn't even know what disease I would be dealing with. In addition, there was a strong clinical component to the research. At ICR I would have the freedom and the funds to organize my research group in the way that I preferred. Even though ICR was dedicated to cancer, we were fundamentally a basic science organization, and we were, at least at that time, never asked what relation our research had to immediate cancer applications.

There was an additional and very practical reason why moving to ICR was advantageous. Before I arrived, Tim Talbot had obtained a grant from the National Cancer Institute, one of the institutes of the NIH, to fund clinical research, but there was no stipulation as to the actual research to be done. We had good funding for staff, equipment, patient care, and all the other necessities, and we could choose the research projects we wished to do. I was in the happy position of being able to decide what I would do without requiring external approval—and the grant was for seven years. Of course, we had to report annually on progress and periodically publish our studies, but we were not required to justify a project and its goals before we actually accomplished them. I have always felt that this was one of the reasons we were able to pursue our work so effectively. We did not have to tell the research review committee what we were going to find before we actually found it. This laid open the possibility for inductive research.

I should add that we subsequently received a supplementary grant for the work we were actually doing—that is, we gained the approval of the research review committee for our particular research—and that it continued to be funded for many years. Another great feature of the move to ICR was that I could hire additional staff of my own choosing to develop what I thought of as clinical research at our center. I will tell you more about my colleagues as the story proceeds.

So I had changed locations, left Washington and Maryland to breathe the salubrious air of the City of Brotherly Love—what happened next? The studies on the sera of transfused patients had been productive. We had found a "new" polymorphism (inherited common biochemical trait) that revealed a rich source of variation in the low-density lipoproteins, an important serum protein involved with diseases of the heart, stroke, and diabetes. But we decided to proceed in another direction in parallel with the research on the lipoprotein polymorphism. Good scientific hypotheses are good because they provide an image of what is happening in nature. They are also good because they generate further hypotheses that lead to interesting experiments that would not otherwise have been devised. At this stage in the work, we placed a greater value on the second use of the model—that is, the rapid generation of new ideas that we would not have imagined without the model. Our minds and hearts were open to any new and interesting discovery.

Since the technique of examining transfused sera had led to the discovery of the antibody that identified the lipoprotein polymorphism, we conjectured that if we continued looking, we would find other precipitating antibodies that would reveal other polymorphisms. Yet the method we used—immunodiffusion in agar gel using the Ouchterlony pattern—manifested both advantages and weaknesses.

First, this method is highly specific. You can determine whether the antigens in different people are the same or different by noting whether the ends of the arcs of precipitation merge with each other or project beyond their juncture. Although more sensitive methods are now available, simple visual examination allowed us to make the same/different distinction. Second, the method is relatively insensitive. In fact, it is one of the least sensitive of the immunological techniques, which are, in general, noted for their great sensitivity. This could be considered a disadvantage, but in the exploratory stage seeing *patterns* of distribution in populations was more important than identifying all possible positives. We decided to continue using immunodiffusion rather than switch to more sensitive methods for detecting antigens, such as radioimmunoassay,[3] that we were even then developing.

---

[3] Radioimmunoassay is a highly sensitive method for identifying specific biochemical and immunological chemicals in biological fluids, using radioactive chemicals as markers.

Third, the immunodiffusion method was inexpensive and could easily be done in the field. It required small (3" × 4") glass plates,[4] agar powder from which gel was made, a metal die to cut out the holes in the gel, and a simple light box to read them. The latter could be improvised with a table lamp and baffle. With our minimal needs, studies could be done anywhere, including laboratories in scientifically underdeveloped countries where expensive equipment was not available. Scientists in the countries where we had worked and where the need for the research was greatest could validate our studies. The simplicity of the method also meant that we could do our studies in a hotel room, on a train, or in an indigenous house without electricity or water in the locations where the blood was actually collected.

Permeating the project was our interest in genetics, inherited susceptibility to disease, and polymorphic systems. This continued even when we realized that we had identified the hepatitis virus. We recognized that there might be a heritable susceptibility to becoming chronically infected, and that this carrier state was a polymorphic system; we could expect a very different responses to infection in different people based on small genetic differences. Some might develop acute responses, from which they readily recovered;others might become chronic carriers of the virus, which could have disease consequences. Our genetics orientation also alerted us to an aspect of infectious diseases that is usually not considered. Polymorphisms may be maintained in a population through a balance of advantages and disadvantages; hence there could be advantages to the carrier state. We had a grand vision of viruses, environmental

---

[4] At the time we were doing these studies, projection slides used in public lectures required 3" by 4" glass plates. Huge electric arc projectors, controlled by professional projectionists, were used to project the slides until about thirty years ago, when 35-mm slide projectors became more common. Ever since, scientific seminars have suffered because of poorly projected slides in machines that typically break down at a crucial moment in the presentation. And it's easy to scramble the small slides when they fall out of the rickety carousels that contain them. A modern scientific speaker has to be prepared to present his talk independent of the order in which the slides are shown.

agents, humans, and other species interacting with one another in a dynamic and complex dance of balanced accommodation.

The Discovery of Australia Antigen during the Search for New Polymorphisms

The American novelist Henry James, in the preface to one of his nonfiction works, uses a delightful metaphor in reference to embarking on a new story:

> *"Roderick Hudson" was my first attempt at a novel, a long fiction with a "complicated" subject, and I recall again the quite uplifted sense with which my idea, such as it was, permitted me at last to put quite out to sea. I had but hugged the shore on sundry previous small occasions; bumping about, to acquire skill, in the shallow waters and sandy coves of the "short story" and master as yet of no vessel constructed to carry a sail. The subject of "Roderick" figured to me vividly this employment of canvas, and I have not forgotten, even after long years, how the blue southern sea seemed to spread immediately before me and the breath of the spice-islands to be already in the breeze.*[5]

We were now venturing out into deep seas and blue water.

A principal goal of science is to provide narrative explanations of natural events. The scientist needs these to synthesize his data, develop concepts, plan new experiments, and, in medicine, identify opportunities for intervention. The public wants explanations to understand the world about them; these stories are a significant product of the scientific enterprise.

Allow me to lay out, in generic form, the ongoing story of discovery of the hepatitis B virus that followed on the discovery of the lipoprotein polymorphism I described in the previous chapter. This may help the reader to follow a narrative that may, at times, seem like a curious mess.

---

[5] H. James, *The Art of the Novel: Critical Prefaces by Henry James*, with an introduction by Richard P. Blackmur (New York: Charles Scribner's Sons, 1934), 4.

We continued to test the general hypothesis that transfused patients would develop antibodies against serum protein antigens they had not inherited. A body of data was generated in the testing of this hypothesis, and antigenic proteins were found. The next step was to use the data to formulate one or more hypotheses—a hypothesis being, to refine our definition, a scientific explanation of the observations, stated in a declarative sentence or sentences, and designed so that the statements are testable by laboratory or observational experiments. In time, we concluded the experiments and evaluated the data to see whether they supported or rejected the hypotheses.

Irrespective of the support or rejection of the hypotheses, we could use the data to formulate one or more new hypotheses. The new hypotheses might be closely related to the original hypothesis or might take off in a completely different direction related to the original hypothesis only by virtue of its having been derived from it. We then decided which of these hypotheses to test; several could be tested more or less simultaneously. The process of hypothesis generation, testing, and formulating new hypotheses continued, but not indefinitely. Eventually, a series of nonrejected hypotheses accumulated, and from these a rather grander vision of the phenomenon was possible: a "big hypothesis," which we may dignify by calling it a "model." This model could now be used to generate a whole new series of hypotheses. At this point it appeared that all we were doing was generating more and more hypotheses, that is, asking a lot of questions. But somewhere in the process it became apparent that a major insight into explanation and application could be derived from this open-ended process. We could see a goal and pursue it with greater direction and precision. We ended up with a large number of answered questions (that is, supported or rejected hypotheses) but also a whole body of untested hypotheses. The amazing thing is that you often don't have to answer all the questions to achieve practical application. Obviously, the more you know, the better equipped you will be to answer questions that arise after application begins.

During 1964, my last year at the National Institutes of Health, we enlarged our studies on the low-density lipoprotein polymorphism.

We also continued the systematic search of sera from patients who had received many transfusions, hoping to find additional antibodies that reacted with other antigenic sites on the low-density lipoprotein molecule. In addition we hoped to find antisera that could identify totally new antigenic polymorphisms among proteins that were not lipoproteins, and thus discover another polymorphic system.

Harvey Alter, a physician member of the clinical and scientific group at the NIH's Blood Bank was one of the many brilliant young physicians who came to work at the institutes in the 1950s and 1960s.[6] Harvey had become interested in our research and was infor-

---

[6] Strangely, this very important contribution to the U.S. effort in basic medical science was, in part, a consequence of the national military conscription laws. After the general conscription of civilians for the U.S. military stopped, the drafting of doctors continued. Military medicine operates on a feast-or-famine basis, to select a particularly inept metaphor. During peacetime, when there are no or few casualties, the potential patient pool is made up of very healthy young men who ordinarily do not require medical care. But when war comes, with its attendant casualties, doctors are needed in large numbers. In readiness for war, which at times seemed imminent, the military had to maintain a large reserve of physicians. However, there were alternatives to conscription into the conventional military forces. The U.S. Public Health Service had been established by Congress shortly after the founding of the federal republic. Its original mission was to supply health care for merchant seamen, sailors who were not in the military but often required medical attention when they landed in U.S. ports that were not their homes. Various duties were added to the charge of the PHS, and in the late nineteenth century Congress designated it a "Uniformed Service." The terms of employment, salary, tenure, and retirement were similar to those of the conventional military forces, and the PHS personnel wore military uniforms while executing many of their functions. During wartime the PHS was militarized, and officers were assigned to duties similar to those that medical officers in the conventional services undertook. (In his excellent scientific autobiography, *For the Love of Enzymes: The Odyssey of a Biochemist* [Cambridge: Harvard University Press, 1989], 7, the Nobel laureate Arthur Kornberg briefly describes his experience as a PHS officer on board a Coast Guard ship during World War II.) Over the years the role of the PHS has changed radically. It is now responsible for the activities at the National Institutes of Health, the Centers for Disease Control, and the Indian Health Services, and for many of the international medical activities of the United States, for the treatment of prisoners in federal penitentiaries, and other duties. Many physicians who had shown a propensity for research were assigned to the laboratories at the National Institutes of Health, and Harvey Alter was one of them.

mally seconded to our laboratory to continue with the work on the sera of transfused patients, many of which were obtained through the Blood Bank. In one of his experiments he saw a precipitin reaction (fig. 1) that was different from the typical lipoprotein bands. The shape of the arc was broader and more graceful, it did not take the lipid stain deeply (indicating that it had less fat than the low-density lipoproteins), and, most important, its distribution in the population was much different from that of the lipoprotein specificities we had identified. The lipoprotein specificities were common (usually more than 50 percent) in most of the populations in which they were tested. However, the newly discovered precipitin was rare; it was not seen in hundreds of sera from the general population of the United States that we tested. But it was found in the sera of people from Taiwan, Vietnam, Korea, the central Pacific, and in several Australian aborigines.

Most of our studies were conducted on the sera from Australians, so we gave the new protein the working name of "Australia antigen," a name that was retained for several years thereafter. A colleague, Dr. Robert Kirk, who was then at the University of Western Australia in Perth, had been conducting studies on the polymorphisms of Australian aborigines, and he had sent the sera to us requesting that we test them for the lipoprotein polymorphic systems. This was a common practice among biochemical population geneticists. A laboratory would specialize in one or more procedures for determining polymorphisms, and people who had collected serum samples would circulate them to the experts to increase the quantity of data gathered on inherited variation for the populations in which they were interested.

Why did we use the name "Australia antigen"? Geographic names are neutral; they make no statement about an inferred hypothesis as to the significance of the phenomenon. When a new protein or other biochemical of potential biological importance is discovered, it is often named to specify its presumed function. This is usually done early in the investigation when only a small fraction of all that could be known is known. Any function that is discovered early in the process probably represents only a part, and possibly not the most biologically relevant part, of the protein's characteris-

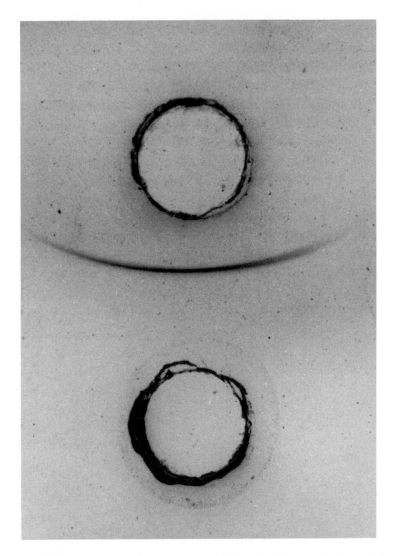

Fig. 1. The first published image of the precipitin reaction in agar gel between Australia antigen and the antibody against it. The precipitin is the combination of the antigen and antibody that forms a visible band in the gel. The top well contains the serum from a patient with leukemia who is a carrier of Australia antigen. The bottom well contains serum from a hemophilia patient who has received many blood transfusions, and contains antibody against Australia antigen. (Blumberg, Alter, and Visnich, *Journal of the American Medical Association* 191 [1965]: 542.)

tics. When a scientist names a new discovery, he has a conscious or subconscious sense of possession and power over the child of his creativity. The name itself is a signature, a mark of possession, but when a scientist discloses his findings by publication or presenting them at a scientific forum, they are no longer private; the discovery belongs to the entire scientific world. The issue is compounded if the scientist, in selecting a name for the new discovery (or creation), implies its function, for then the scientist's ego is wrapped up in not only the name but also the biological activity of the substance. When testing the hypothesis of function, the experimenter may be biased in favor of the original explanation, and this could hamper objective evaluation of data. Therein lies one of the great dangers of the scientific process, the abandonment of unbiased judgment in the service of self.

The antibody that was used to find Australia antigen came from a hemophilia patient from New York City who had received many transfusions.[7] We discovered that transfused hemophilia patients often had the antibody and were a major resource for the reagents used in the research. We did not work immediately on the new antigen, as we had a great deal to do on the lipoprotein polymorphism project, but we did not forget it. This pattern is not uncommon in research. New data flow in, and at the time it is hard to determine which of the possible directions is the best to follow. That evaluation can be made only after the outcome is known. But when you're living it, you don't know what the future will bring. Nor do you know what the outcome of testing the other hypotheses would have wrought. Scientists have a strange sense of possible parallel worlds—depending on which hypothesis is tested—and ordinarily they will never know the outcome of the undone experiment.

---

[7] Hemophilia is a disorder in which proteins needed to form a blood clot are missing or reduced. This can result in uncontrollable bleeding episodes that result in the need for many transfusions. In addition, patients are often given replacement protein, antihemophilia globulin, prepared from the blood of many donors. For these reasons, hemophilia patients are exposed to sera from a very large number of individuals and are likely to become infected with blood-borne agents, or to develop antibodies against serum proteins.

I'm often asked why we were testing sera from Australian aborigines. The answer derives from our overriding interest in human inherited variation—polymorphisms. Our long-term goal in studying what at that time was an esoteric field in human population genetics was to find relations between these polymorphisms and differences in susceptibility to disease. We knew that the frequency of polymorphic alleles varies greatly from population to population and from country to country. In looking for a new polymorphism without any knowledge of the population distribution of the alleles, we reckoned that we could increase the probability of success by randomizing the populations used in the screens of the transfused sera. Consequently, in each of the test panels we included sera from different populations, and the screen in which the new antiserum was found included, not exactly by chance, Australian aborigines.

I had reviewed this notion in several of our early papers and expressed it again in an address, later published, that I gave as the Fifth Bernadine Becker Memorial Lecture of the New York Rheumatism Society,[8] which, if I recall correctly, was not well attended. I said:

> As a consequence of disease and environmental forces as well as other factors, a large number of polymorphisms may exist in a population. Some may be related to present selective forces and others to forces which operated in the past, but which are no longer significant.

The study of inherited variation was basic, non-goal-directed research designed to illuminate a natural biological phenomenon. In medical research, or for that matter any form of fundamental research, there is a belief—one might even say faith—that knowledge and understanding although not immediately useful will, in the end, lead to practical application.

It was in the published version of the Becker Lecture that mention was first made in print of the newly discovered inherited antigen

---

[8] B. S. Blumberg, "Iso-antibodies in Humans against Inherited Serum Low Density Beta-lipoproteins, the Ag System," *Annals of the New York Academy of Sciences* 103 (1963): 1052–57.

we subsequently called Australia antigen, and which drew us away, at least temporarily, from the pure pursuit of polymorphic traits. Now, the question was "What is this Australia antigen?" We were in the same position as when we first found the antibody in the blood of Mr. C. deB. and didn't know the protein it reacted with. In the case of Australia antigen the question was just as perplexing and the answer was very different.

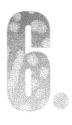 ## What Is Australia Antigen?

WE STARTED our new search on the assumption that Australia antigen (Au) was also an inherited protein. But it soon became clear that it had additional very interesting characteristics; we experienced a "Eureka" event, so often described in the annals of scientific discovery. In our case, it wasn't exactly a single leap but a series of gradually unfolding events.

We initially discovered the "Ag system" using the technique of immunodiffusion with transfused sera as the source of antibody. The next discovery was the Australia antigen, which we continued to follow and which I will describe in this chapter. But we also discovered other antibodies in the sera from the transfused patients that we pursued for a relatively short time. The "Pennsylvania antigen" was the subject of at least one published paper. The results were inconclusive, and we discontinued the project. Antisera against antigens we called Hu, Fx, Tx, and others were found; some of these appeared to be directed against *Pseudomonas* bacteria, but this project was also discontinued.

Were these antisera, other than Ag and Au, blind alleys? Why did we continue with Australia antigen and not with the others? How would we know those others were blind alleys if we didn't follow through the research? If we had persevered, they might have led to other findings possibly as interesting and useful as those that resulted from the Australia antigen lead. The decision to pursue a given research path is often rationally based, but sometimes it is a question of intuition—a kind of wisdom that you possess but can't articulate to yourself or to others. The most likely reason for our continuing with Au and not the other antisera is that we had discovered it earlier. We built up a significant body of data that looked promising, the reagents were available, and the experiments were reproducible. Another possibility is that we were lucky in deciding on this line of inquiry; I am quite prepared to accept this explanation. But, like the speaker of Robert Frost's famous poem, I still wonder where the other paths in the woods would have gone.

To continue with the Australia antigen studies, we had to obtain more data to formulate additional hypotheses that would get us on the track of illuminating the subject. During 1964 we started a systematic study of the disease and geographic distribution of Au. The antigen was stable in frozen serum. We had saved and frozen the blood collected while we were studying inherited biochemical variation, and we were able to do an extensive survey of many populations from different parts of the world in a relatively short time (see table 1). Au was rare in normal U.S. populations but common in Asia, the Pacific, Africa, and eastern and southern Europe. These very first studies showed us the populations where the prevalence of Au and, as we later learned, of carriers of HBV was high. They pointed to where the public health problems were greatest, and where I would be doing my field trips for several decades to come.

The initial studies also revealed familial clustering of Au. It is not surprising that we had looked at families; our previous research on biochemical polymorphisms required that we study families to determine whether the traits were inherited. By chance, the first of our family studies was done in a small and ancient—in fact, biblical—population. How this came about is in many ways typical of the apparently random and fortuitous manner in which research collaborations develop, and in which apparently unrelated activities are brought together.

Dr. Batsheva Bonné, a serological geneticist and anthropologist from Israel, was visiting our laboratory. She had been involved in a detailed investigation of the biochemical polymorphisms of the small population of Samaritans living in Israel, and was in the process of determining the prevalence of the alleles of the low-density

TABLE 1
**The Distribution of Au in Various Populations, as
Reported in the Initial Studies**

Population	No. Tested	Australia Antigen Present	
		No.	%
Aborigines, Australia	208	12	6
Chinese, USA, and Taiwan	65	0	0
Eskimo, Alaska	24	0	0
Greeks, Greece	179	8	4
Indians, Canada	78	0	0
Indians, Mexico	100	1	1
Israelis	96	2	2
Japanese, USA	48	0	0
Koreans	1	1	
Micronesians, Rongelap	193	7	4
African American, USA	241	0	0
Newborn children, white	18	0	0
Polynesians, Bora Bora	24	1	4
Samaritans, Israel	125	2	2
Taiwanese	23	3	13
Tristan da Cunha Islanders	42	0	0
Vietnamese	24	1	4
White, USA	215	0	0
Total	1,704	38	

Source: Blumberg, Alter, and Visnick, *Journal of the American Medical Association* 191 (1965): 543.

lipoprotein polymorphism.[1] Batsheva tested 125 of the sera for Au. Two were positive; they were siblings who were the offspring of a cousin marriage.[2] Because of the small size of the population and the desire to maintain cultural homogeneity, cousin marriages were common among the Samaritans.

[1] The Samaritans are a community, then resident in Israel and Jordan, who claim descent from the Jews of ancient Samaria who remained in the Holy Land when the majority of the Jewish population were exiled to Babylon by the Assyrian conquerors of Israel in 772 B.C. Their Bible included only the five books of Moses and not the remainder of the canon.

[2] B. S. Blumberg, H. J. Alter, and S. Visnich, "A 'New' Antigen in Leukemia Sera," *Journal of the American Medical Association* 191 (1965): 541–46.

During the 1960s we continued the family studies. They were based mainly on field trips (starting in 1965) to Cebu in the Visayan Islands group in the central Philippines, a few hundred miles south of Manila. Why Cebu? It's a long story, but the short version is that the Leonard Wood[3] Memorial of the American Leprosy Foundation had, for many years, maintained a Hansen's disease (leprosy)[4] hospital, clinic, and research laboratory on the island. Dr. Michel Lechat[5] was conducting a study on polymorphic traits associated with the different clinical forms of leprosy. We were assisting with these studies and were given permission to look for Au in the population. There was a high frequency of Au in this population, and we learned that it would be possible to collect biological material from families that were being studied as a consequence of the leprosy genetics project. Additionally, we had families from other locations in the Pacific and South America. Formally, the hypothesis to be tested stated that individuals homozygous[6] for a gene designated Au^1 (i.e.,

---

[3] Leonard Wood had a remarkable medical and military career. While an assistant surgeon with the Army during the Apache Campaign of 1886 he won the Medal of Honor. During the Spanish-American War, he was the commander of the First Volunteer Cavalry ("Rough Riders"); Theodore Roosevelt was his second in command. He fought in the Philippines in 1904 during the bloody battles following the Spanish-American War. President Taft—who had known him in the Philippines, where Taft had served as the civilian governor—later named him Army chief of staff. In 1921 he was appointed governor-general of the Philippines; during this period he became interested in the plight of the Hansen's disease patients common in the country at the time. He encouraged the establishment of an organization for research and treatment of leprosy, and, following his death in 1927, the Leonard Wood Memorial was established in his honor.

[4] The current designation for leprosy is Hansen's disease, after the Norwegian physician who is credited with the first modern description. This name has been used to remove some of the opprobrium attached to the disease even in contemporary society.

[5] Dr. Lechat had been a medical officer at a large leprosarium in the Congo, when it was still a colony of Belgium. Graham Greene, the British novelist, visited Michel's leprosarium at Iyonda, Equator Province, when he was researching his novel *A Burnt-Out Case* (1960; New York: Penguin USA, 1992). He dedicated the book to Michel and made him the model for the novel's heroic medical doctor.

[6] "Homozygous" means that the same allele was inherited from both the mother and the father. In heterozygotes different genes are inherited from each of the parents.

genotype Au^1/Au^1) have detectable Australia antigen in their blood. They are phenotype Au(1). Individuals homozygous for the alternative allele, Au, whose product was not known (Au/Au), or heterozygotes (Au^1 / Au) do not have detectable Australia antigen. They are phenotype Au(0). The family data we had collected were consistent with this model.

We were mindful that the genetic pattern of distribution did not rule out an infectious cause. In the paper in which we first described Australia antigen, we had included the hypothesis that Au was a virus found in the blood of the leukemia patients and other individuals who had tested positive. However, both the genetic and viral hypotheses were tenable. Later, when we realized that Au was part of the hepatitis B virus, we changed our model to state that there was an inherited *susceptibility* to becoming a persistent carrier. Individuals who had inherited certain alleles would be relatively susceptible to chronic infection, and those who had inherited alternative alleles would be relatively resistant. If the person were not infected with HBV, then the pattern of inheritance would not be revealed. But in regions of the world where HBV was pervasive, most individuals who had inherited the hypothesized susceptibility gene or genes (Au^1) would, if infected, become carriers, and the pattern of Mendelian inheritance would be evident. However, not everyone who was susceptible would be exposed, and as a consequence there would not be 100 percent "penetrance,"[7]—that is, the Mendelian ratios would not be exactly fulfilled.

Subsequent studies by other investigators cast doubt on the initial genetic conclusions because there were exceptions to the expected segregation in the families. Many years later, my friend and colleague Edward Lustbader completed more sophisticated analyses that also supported the inheritance model.[8] In any case, we decided that we had little to gain in continuing the classical family

[7] If the product of the gene is always present when the gene or genes are present, the gene is said to be "100 percent penetrant." Percentages less than 100 give the probability that the effect of the gene can be detected.

[8] Ed Lustbader was the statistician for our group for many years and had a big impact on the design and interpretation of most of our experiments. Sadly, he died in 1996 at age forty-nine of cancer, ironically, the disease to whose understanding he

segregation studies; they did not seem to impress our colleagues, and doing more of them was unlikely to have much of an effect. We realized that we had to wait until more was known about the genes and the molecular biology of HBV before we could proceed. That took a few years.

How We Arrived at the Hypothesis That Australia Antigen Was Part of a Hepatitis Virus

A series of "background" events led to the generation of the hypothesis that Au was part of the hepatitis virus. In research, important ideas do not often spring up in isolation like Aphrodite suddenly rising from the sea, incompletely clothed, and served up on a scallop shell.[9] Usually a lengthy period of observations and ideas forms a background of knowledge. Into this mix may fall a particularly crucial piece (or, more often, pieces) of information, which, like a seed cast into well-manured and cultivated soil, grows and flourishes. Darwin's concept of evolution did not come in a sudden insightful flash. He was greatly influenced by evolutionary ideas about geology that derived from his mentor Lyell, whose books he read aboard the *Beagle*. He carried the first volume out with him from England, and the second reached him on the Pacific coast of Chile soon after he had seen the uplifted strata in southern South America that also influenced his evolutionary thinking. Another factor was the great verse tome embodying notions of evolution that his grandfather, Erasmus Darwin, had written. Charles Darwin's own comparison of the different stages in the evolution of coral formations—fringing reefs, atolls, and barrier reefs—published before his book on his theory of evolution, also prepared him for the concept of evolutionary change in nature.

---

had contributed greatly over the span of his career. His genetic analysis has not yet been published.

[9] This may not be such a great metaphor. Those of you familiar with the unusual turns of Greek myths will recall that Aphrodite/Venus actually arose from the foam produced by the severed genitals of an incestuous father.

Scientists may perceive that great concepts *can* strike suddenly in a fit of instant revelation. There are well-known examples of this. Alfred Russel Wallace (1823–1913), the coauthor with Darwin of the theory of evolution, claimed that the idea came to him in 1858 during a bout of malarial fever at Ternate in the Moluccas (now Indonesia), where he was collecting butterflies:

> I was suffering from a sharp attack of intermittent fever, and every day during the cold and succeeding hot fits had to lie down for several hours, during which time I had nothing to do but to think over any subject then particularly interesting to me. . . . Why do some die and some live? And the answer was clearly, that on the whole the best fitted live. From the effects of disease the most healthy escaped; from enemies, the strongest, the swiftest or the most cunning; from famine, the best hunters or those with the best digestion; and so on. that is, the fittest would survive. . . . I awaited anxiously for the termination of my fit so that I might at once make notes for a paper on the subject.[10]

Friedrich August Kekule von Stradonitz (1829–96), who discovered the ring structure for benzene, said that the concept took shape during a dream when he saw a snake with its tail in its mouth.

> My mental eye, rendered more acute by repeated visions of the kind, could now distinguish larger structures of manifold conformation: long rows, sometimes more closely fitted together all twining and twisting in snake-like motion. But look! What was that? One of the snakes had seized hold of its own tail, and the form whirled mockingly before my eyes. As if by a flash of lightning I awoke; and this time also I spent the rest of the night in working out the consequences of the hypothesis.[11]

But even in the case of these epiphany moments, there is surely a complex background to the scientific discovery.

In our case the series of observations and experiments may not have been as dramatic as the classical examples I have cited, but they served nonetheless to create a background for our formulating the hypothesis that Au was part of a hepatitis virus. The process

---

[10] A. R. Wallace, *My Life* (London: Chapman & Hall, 1905).
[11] O. T. Benfey, *Journal of Chemical Education* 35 (1958): 22.

proceeded in the following sequence. First, there were a series of observations—some casual, others generated during the testing of hypotheses—that gradually heightened our suspicion that we were dealing with a virus that caused hepatitis. This in turn led to the hypothesis that Au would be found more frequently in patients with hepatitis than in controls. This was tested in clinical studies and validated. Finally, we tested, and supported, the hypothesis that Au *was* a hepatitis virus or was located on it.

Many scientists did these studies over the course of the next ten years or more. We worked as a coherent unit of Fox Chase Cancer Center—the Division of Clinical Research—and stayed together for most of the project. More information about my coworkers is included in Appendix 1 at the end of the book.

Now, to the details of the story.

From our studies in the United States of what appeared to be a random selection of patients (1964–65), we saw that most of the sera containing Au were from patients who had been transfused. This was probably our first inkling that Au might be a blood-transmitted infectious agent. In my "General Notes" for November 1965 I recorded that we had discussed transfusion studies, an indication that we were thinking about a blood-transmitted agent. This was followed by another apparently random observation that again tipped our thinking to hepatitis. As part of our survey of normal populations, we tested sera that had been sent to us by an unusual figure in the research community. Curtis Hames was a general practitioner in Claxton, a rural community in Evans County in southern Georgia. Based on his own practice and access to the whole population of the county irrespective of their ability to pay, he established a long-term population-based study of cardiovascular disease. By "population-based" I mean that he looked not only at patients but at nonhospitalized people who might be at risk. He used modern laboratory and clinical methods, in part by calling on his academic collaborators, and established one of the most comprehensive studies on medical, social, dietary, and other factors that contribute to the risk of cardiovascular disease. He made his resources available to others doing population studies as long as they did not additionally inconvenience his study subjects. We had helped him in the past by determining the distribution of polymorphisms along the lines discussed in the earlier chapters. He allowed us to use the same blood specimens, obtained from apparently healthy members of the community, as part of our project to determine the distribution of Au in the general population.

In 1966 we tested several hundred of the Evans County sera and found that only one was positive for Au. We were, of course, curious to know whether there was anything that distinguished this person from all the others who did not have Au. I called Curt on the phone to tell him our finding, and he said he would get back to me if he learned anything of importance. I soon heard from him again; the person with Au was, in fact, not part of the normal population study, but one of his patients who had been diagnosed with hepatitis! This again raised our level of suspicion, but at the time it was just one more piece of data crowding into our more or less overloaded brains along with many other bits.

Yet another apparently casual observation in "normal" persons raised our background sensitivity to hepatitis. We had been allowed to test the blood, collected for a health survey, of the employees of a large organization. We did this anonymously—that is, the names of the individuals tested were disassociated from the code markings on the tubes holding the specimens. Of more than a thousand tested specimens, only one was found to be positive. We subsequently learned that this person had received a blood transfusion a short time before the blood had been collected. Again, a small tweak in our consciousness that an infectious agent might have been transmitted via the blood.

A few other clues were contributed as a consequence of the hypothesis testing that emerged from the initial set of observations. We designed these hypotheses to gain straightforward information concerning the character and distribution of the Australia antigen. For example, was the antigen persistent in the blood? That is, if it was present at one point in time, would it be present when it was subsequently tested? This information is usually required when scientists study what is thought to be an inherited trait. The biochemical product of a gene is usually, but not always, present for a long period after its first appearance. To test the persistence hypothesis for Au, we obtained serial samples of blood from people with and without Au. We tested this notion no fewer than twelve times in patients with thalassemia (a hemoglobin synthesis disorder) from Italy, in renal dialysis patients from Philadelphia, and in others. In general, we found support for the hypothesis that the presence of Au was persistent, but there were interesting exceptions, and I will describe two important examples.

In November 1967 we evaluated the results of a study of sera that had been collected over time from inhabitants of Rongelap Atoll in the Pacific Marshall Islands. This population was being surveyed in yearly follow-up studies subsequent to their exposure to radiation on 1 March 1954 as a result of the detonation of a nuclear device during the Bravo test on Bikini Atoll in the U.S. Trust Territories of the Pacific Islands. There have been many scientific reports on these victims, and even more writing on the human, social, and political consequences of the testing.[12] As part of the health survey, we tested sequential specimens collected from the same individual over the course of several years. One of the tested persons had an interesting sequence of results. In 1964 he had no detectable Au precipitins. In 1965 he received a single blood transfusion for the treatment of a bleeding ulcer, after which he had antibody against Au. The next year, the antibody had disappeared and Australia antigen was present. This again raised the possibility of an infectious agent transmitted by blood because antibodies often form in people who have been infected. Although this observation piqued our interest, some time elapsed before we could fit it properly into the infectious model.

The incident that made the biggest impression on us occurred under our very eyes. Again, it was a consequence of testing the per-

---

[12] The Brookhaven National Laboratory has periodically published the results of the medical survey. See, for example, R. A. Conard, L. M. Meyer, W. W. Sutow, B. S. Blumberg, A. Lowery, S. H. Cohn, W. H. Lewis, Jr., J. W. Hollingsworth, and H. W. Lyon, *Medical Survey of Rongelap People Five and Six Years after Exposure to Fallout* (Brookhaven National Laboratory, 1960).

sistence hypothesis, this time in patients with Down's syndrome.[13] How did this study come about? To put it in an appropriate conceptual framework, I will return to a set of hypotheses generated from the data on the distribution of Au in different populations and under different circumstances. We found that Au was rare in normal U.S. populations but common in some disease groups. The most striking finding was its high prevalence in patients with leukemia. This dichotomy allowed for several interesting, if simplistic, hypotheses. One was that Au was the cause of leukemia and was related to the viruses that at that time were thought to be the cause of one or more human leukemias.[14] Another hypothesis was that leukemia generated the Au in the blood. A third possibility was that there was a common cause—for example, a genetic trait that led to both the development of leukemia *and* the presence of Au. We started testing all three hypotheses. It was simpler and faster to test the third by testing a corollary, namely, that individuals who were at high risk of developing leukemia were more likely to have a high prevalence of Au.

We could identify several groups at high risk for leukemia. It was an interesting list: it included residents of Hiroshima and Nagasaki who had been within a thousand meters of ground zero at the time the nuclear weapons were dropped on their cities in 1945, and who had survived. Strange as it may seem, detailed information about these populations was available. Shortly after the end of the war a group of scientists went to Hiroshima and Nagasaki to study the survivors of the first (and, so far, only) victims of nuclear war. The Atomic Bomb Casualty Commission, the name of this research orga-

---

[13] Down's syndrome is a common form of mental retardation associated with, in most cases, the presence of three copies of chromosome 21. The overall incidence is about 1/700 births, but in mothers over forty it is 1/40, a very high risk. Older pregnant women are often screened to determine whether they are carrying a Down's syndrome child. The patients have a low IQ, around 50, but usually a very pleasant and loving personality. There are other physical abnormalities, including a high prevalence of heart disease and susceptibility to acute leukemia.

[14] This belief arose in large part from the observation that mouse, cat, and other animal leukemias were caused by specific viruses.

nization, was first administered by the military, then by the Atomic Energy Commission, and later, when nuclear weapons were subsumed under "energy," by the newly created Department of Energy. In 1975 the ABCC was superseded by the Radiation Effect Research Foundation, a Japanese organization, but still operated with the cooperation of U.S. scientists.[15] A detailed census was taken, estimates were made of the probable radiation dose each person had been subjected to, and a program for medical follow-up and research was initiated that has continued for more than fifty years. I visited the Hiroshima headquarters of the ABCC in 1967 during the course of a field trip to Japan and the Philippines, and asked the scientists at the site whether they (or we) could test the sera of the people who were resident in the city at the time of the bombing. They were unable do the studies then. Several years later they did report that the frequency of Au in the population was related to the amount of radiation exposure, as we had predicted.

A second group with a high risk of leukemia were patients with ankylosing spondylitis[16] who had been treated with X ray. We eventually obtained sera from such patients, but we did not find an increased prevalence of Au. In this case the predictive power of the hypothesis was not good. A third group were patients with Down's syndrome, who have a higher likelihood of developing leukemia

[15] Further information on this organization can be obtained at website www.eml.doe.gov/hsrd/hsr95/nas.htm

[16] Ankylosing spondylitis is an uncommon form of arthritis that affects the sacroiliac joint and the intervertebral discs of the spine. It results in a bent spine; in advanced cases, the curvature of the spine can be extreme. Sometimes the neck vertebrae are fused so that it is difficult for the patient to turn his or her head. Other investigators showed that if the patients had been irradiated as part of their treatment, which was a common practice, they had an increased risk for leukemia. I knew a lot about this disease because I had written a comprehensive clinical review of the cases when, in 1956, I was a fellow in the Department of Medicine at Columbia-Presbyterian Medical Center. (B. S. Blumberg and C. Ragan, "The Natural History of Rheumatoid Spondylitis," *Medicine* 35 [1956]: 1–31.) Bernard Connor (or O'Connor), a seventeenth-century Irish physician and scientist, published the first clinical description of the disease. My wife and I wrote a historical monograph about him, and, as a consequence of my enthusiasm, my first son has Connor as a middle name.

than normal children or than mentally retarded children without Down's syndrome. In the event, the Down's syndrome group was the most interesting. First, some deep background about the patients.

Contemporary practice is to encourage caring for mentally retarded children in the family home, or in small institutions, but this was not the case in the 1960s. Mentally retarded and mentally ill patients were for the most part retained in large institutions usually run by state health departments. When I was in medical school in the late 1940s, we were instructed to tell the parents of mentally retarded children that their offspring should be placed in the care of the community early in life, before the parents became too attached to their disabled children. How different from current attitudes! Doctors in the 1960s learned nothing about mental retardation; this was the province of the social workers and special education people (of whom there were few), and doctors were expected to be involved with more curable conditions.

The state institutions for the mentally retarded had thousands of inpatients and were often in remote rural locations. It was as if society wanted to rid itself of disabled people who were a difficult challenge to their collective humanity. In later years when I did fieldwork in institutions for leprosy patients, I could not help but notice the similarity in the public's disregard for these unfortunate patient groups. Traditionally leprosy—Hansen's disease—patients had been segregated and kept away from population centers, and it appeared that the mentally retarded were regarded in the same opprobrious light. Because these institutions were large and unwieldy, and because they were very expensive to administer, they often did not have sufficient resources. There were recurrent scandals and exposés about what was said to be poor care and even inhumane treatment. However, at the institutions where we worked in New Jersey and Pennsylvania, I was very impressed with the quality, the concern, and the dedication of the administration and staff.

After obtaining an introduction to the director of the institution, we attended meetings of the parents association to tell them what we planned to do, and to obtain their agreement and permission. We would draw blood, in some cases in connection with a public health or clinical program that would be of immediate value to the residents. At the time we did the study, we did not know we were detecting hepatitis virus, as we were still testing the hypothesis that led to this conclusion. I explained to the parents that the study was not of immediate relevance to their children, but that if it did prove to have clinical importance, the children who participated in the study would be among the first to be offered any advantage that derived from it. It was very gratifying to our research group when, several years later and after the vaccine had been invented and developed, Down's syndrome patients were among the early beneficiaries of the vaccination program.[17]

We observed the patients in the institution and at our hospital in Philadelphia. Our study was designed to test the hypothesis that Au would be more common in Down's children than in mentally retarded patients with other diagnoses. Remember that it was the Down's syndrome patients who were known to have an increased risk of leukemia. The results of the studies were very exciting; I can recall looking at the experiments as they unfolded in the laboratory. The test panel sera were placed in the peripheral wells of the Ouchterlony plate, and the serum from the transfused person in the center well. If the serum was "positive"—that is, contained Au—a beautiful arc of precipitation appeared between the center well containing the antiserum against Au and the peripheral well containing the serum to be tested. The experiments were set out one morning, and usually by the next day they were ready for reading. We saw many bands on the plate, and when the results were decoded and arrayed in a table, there were far more positives in the Down's syndrome patients than in the controls, as we had predicted.

There is something magical about hypothesis testing. The outcome of the experiment is predicted on the basis of previous observation and theoretical knowledge. In effect, you are stating what will happen in the future; you are a prophet. The sense of power, of control, is heady, but for the experienced scientist it is tempered by

[17] An interesting discussion of the problem of Down's syndrome patients and hepatitis is given in W. Muraskin, "Individual Rights versus the Public Health: The Controversy over the Integration of Retarded Hepatitis B Children into the New York City Public School System," *Journal of the History of Medicine and Allied Sciences* 45 (1990): 64–98.

the knowledge that future predictions made on the basis of the same hypothesis may not be accurate. Having said that, I cherish the moments and enjoy the happiness that comes with discovery. There is also a special pleasure in sharing the experience of discovery with others. At my laboratory, we were a close-knit "Corps of Discovery"—that's the phrase Lewis and Clark, the American army explorers, used to describe their expedition to the Pacific—and it was great to share the excitement with my colleagues as the results of the Down's study flowed in.

In line with our practice of testing and retesting a hypothesis in different situations, we decided to continue the investigation in other institutions for the mentally retarded. We tested the hypothesis that Au would be common in Down's syndrome patients again in large institutions in Pennsylvania and in the state of Washington. It was supported in both. At about the time we were doing our studies, mentally retarded patients were beginning to be withdrawn from large establishments and housed in small units of a few dozen or even smaller numbers in houses and institutions in the community. We studied several of these smaller patient populations, and here we found that the antigen was either absent or in much lower frequency than it had been in the larger institutions. Formally, this finding ruled against our hypothesis. Actually, we were quite satisfied that the multiple studies we had done in the large institutions were valid, particularly because they supported each other and were based on substantial numbers. But the small-institution results led us to the formulation of a new hypothesis, namely, that there was a factor, inversely related to institution size, that decreased the frequency of Au in the Down's patients in the small units. It did not take a great leap of intelligence for us to recognize that the prevalence of Au could be due to an infectious process. Infections of many kinds are more readily transmitted in large institutions, particularly where it is not possible to maintain high standards of sanitation. This observation added to our growing belief that we were dealing with an infectious agent. The Down's syndrome patients, whom we were observing over the course of time, also provided another group in whom we could test the persistence hypothesis, and these observations were crucial in our discovery process.

Australia Antigen and the Hepatitis Virus

One of our patients from the institution for the mentally retarded in New Jersey, James Bair,[18] had several sequential tests that were negative. Then, contrary to our expectation, his blood tested positive. James was admitted to our research unit for more intensive clinical study. Most serum proteins are produced in the liver, and since one of our hypotheses was that Au was caused by disease, we did a series of "liver function" tests to determine whether any pathological changes had occurred. They had. Alton Sutnick, a senior physician in our group who was responsible for James's medical care, wrote in the patient's chart on 28 June 1966:

> SGOT slightly elevated! Prothrombin time low! We may have an indication of [the reason for] his conversion to Au+.[19]

The clinical chemistry results were consistent with a mild case of hepatitis. We inferred that James had developed the liver disease between the time he had been negative and the time he became positive. This was another "hint," and a strong one, that Au was associated with hepatitis.

This observation energized our interest in testing the hypothesis that Au was associated with hepatitis. Our collection of sera from

---

[18] Ordinarily, patients in clinical studies are treated anonymously, or only initials or numbers are used. But James and his parents have become caught up in this project, and the Bairs not only allowed us to identify their son but urged us to do so. When James was born, it was the practice to advise parents to place their children under custodial care. This was the case with James, but his parents, who had moved away from New Jersey to the Midwest, kept in close contact with their son. We maintained our contacts with them during and after his hospitalization, and for many years afterward we would see Mr. and Mrs. Bair during their visits to James. They told us they were pleased that their son had played an important role in the discovery of HBV, and that his involvement as a study subject had favorably influenced the health of so many other people. It had provided some small counterbalance to the difficulty they had encountered after the birth of a mentally retarded child.

[19] The *SGOT* is an enzyme present in liver cells. When the cells are damaged by disease, the enzyme leaks out into the blood and can be detected. *Prothrombin* is a protein manufactured in the liver that is involved in blood clotting. When the liver

patients with the diagnosis of clinical hepatitis accelerated. By mid-1967, we had collected and tested a sufficient number of sera to determine that the frequency of Au was significantly elevated in the patients with acute hepatitis. (We later also found a strong association with chronic hepatitis.) We wrote a paper describing our findings and conclusions and submitted it to the *Annals of Internal Medicine*. To our great disappointment, the paper was returned. The editor informed us that it was not acceptable for publication; the reviewers felt that we had not convincingly supported our hypothesis.

The rejection was off-putting, as it was a message that the research community was not as convinced of the validity of our studies as we were. This is not uncommon in medical research; if such rejections are taken too seriously, they can lead to an attitude of martyrdom and of opposition to a recalcitrant establishment. The editor of the *Annals*, Ed Huth, later told me that he thought that the rejection of our paper was one of the big errors of judgment the journal had made. On several occasions after the event and after our finding had been amply confirmed, Dr. Gerald Klatskin, the reviewer who actually rejected the paper, confessed that he had deemed ours to be just one more in a series of reports claiming that the hepatitis virus had been found. In his experience, previous findings had been subsequently refuted when tested by other investigators. He didn't want to risk another false claim for the identification of the elusive virus; and, erring on the side of caution, he had recommended the rejection of our article.

We may have harbored unhappy sentiments for a while, but they didn't last, and the rebuff didn't slow us down. At about the time the main paper was rejected, an earlier paper submitted to the same journal had been accepted, and it included our initial observations on the Au-hepatitis association. This paper was published in 1967.[20] In earlier papers we had suggested that Au might be associated with a virus, but in the 1967 paper we definitively stated that Au could

is malfunctioning, its levels decrease. In the Sutnick quotation, the words in brackets are added. The exclamation points are not.

[20] B. S. Blumberg, B.J.S. Gerstley, D. A. Hungerford, W. T. London, and A. I. Sutnick, "A Serum Antigen (Australia Antigen) in Down's Syndrome Leukemia and Hepatitis," *Annals of Internal Medicine* 66 (1967): 924–31.

be associated with a hepatitis virus. We had released the genie from the bottle, and big things began to happen.

One of the most important steps we took was to distribute vials of the antiserum and the antigen to investigators who requested it. With these, it was very easy for scientists, even in laboratories with rudimentary equipment, to repeat and extend our studies. Within a few months there was confirmation from other investigators, often from parts of the world where hepatitis B was more common than in the United States. Among them was Professor Kazuo Okochi, then at the University of Tokyo. Alberto Vierruci in Siena, Italy, also published one of the early confirmations. Alfred Prince[21] at the New York Blood Bank studied U.S. patients and emphasized that the virus we had identified was analogous to the posttransfusion hepatitis virus that had been inferred from the earlier research in the field. In time, the virus associated with Au was designated as hepatitis B. This term had been introduced before we discovered the virus, when its existence was still hypothetical. It served to distinguish the blood-transmitted agent B from hepatitis A, which was hypothesized to be transmitted by the fecal-oral route (i.e., by people's eating or drinking the waste of other humans).

The Nature of Scientific Revolutions

We had, unexpectedly, entered the realm of hepatitis research—a field with a long history that, until now, we had not shared. References to yellow jaundice, the signature symptom of hepatitis, had appeared in early sources, for example, the Babylonian Talmud (about A.D. 200 to 500). The Hippocratic writers and, particularly, Galen wrote detailed clinical descriptions of jaundice and started the unraveling of the various causes of this symptom. Pope Zacharias (later Saint Zachary) was said to have recognized, in the eighth century, the infectious nature of jaundice and to have

---

[21] Initially, there was an assertion that the virus reported by Prince was different from ours, but this was later resolved when it became apparent that the two were essentially the same.

recommended the isolation of cases. Epidemics were described as early as the eighteenth century in Geneva, Minorca, Mainz, and many other locations. By the mid–nineteenth century, the reports were numerous, particularly of military outbreaks. It is now known that, in addition to viruses, the causes of jaundice include diseases that break down the red blood cells (for example, sickle-cell diseases), parasites that infect the liver, and acute and chronic liver disease caused by alcohol and other liver toxins. Cancer that originates in the liver and cancer that spreads to the liver from other organs can also lead to clinical jaundice.

Perhaps we should have been more annoyed when our initial paper on the association between hepatitis and Au was not accepted for publication. We were disappointed that the "establishment" did not readily accept our findings. But their reaction was quite understandable. Many scientists had been working on this problem intensively for years. We were not part of this group; none of us was a virologist, we had not been formally trained as epidemiologists, nor did we have any special expertise as hepatitis clinicians beyond our ordinary experience as physicians. My previous research had concerned arthritis and human population genetics. Nor did the other members of the group have prior involvement with hepatitis. Tom London had worked in endocrinology and the epidemiology of thyroid disease. Alton Sutnick was a cardiologist and had studied biochemicals that line the respiratory passages. Irving Millman was the only one of us with graduate training in microbiology, and his main interest had been in tuberculosis and other bacteria. We found the hepatitis virus while we were looking at quite different things. We were outsiders not known to the main body of hepatitis investigators, some of whom had been pursuing their field of interest for decades.

We were surprised at the apparent hostility occasionally engendered among our new colleagues. I eventually realized what was going on when I read Thomas Kuhn's *The Structure of Scientific Revolutions*,[22] which had recently been published and was making a big impact on the thinking about scientific process. Kuhn's thesis—or,

---

[22] T. S. Kuhn, *The Structure of Scientific Revolutions* (Chicago: University of Chicago Press, 1962).

to be more accurate, my perception of it—is that science progresses in a series of revolutionary steps. In a given field of science, the established practitioners, the high priests of the discipline or subdiscipline, have a model that defines the main principles of agreed-upon and accepted belief. Kuhn used the term "paradigm," which has a greater weight or dignity than "model" or "hypothesis." A paradigm is a grand version of these, such as the theory of evolution, or germ theory, or the heliocentric universe, or atomic/molecular structure—big stuff. "Paradigm" became a buzzword, useful at social gatherings of nonscientists as well as in scientific circles. The paradigm is learned at the master's knee; it is the revealed wisdom that students receive from their mentors, and carries with it the connotation of authority, incorporating respect for the elders from whom the younger scientists derived their training.

Because of the great measure of respect it commands, the paradigm is not easily dislodged. If small arrows seem to hit the mark and erode the paradigm, then small changes may be made to accommodate the insistent new knowledge. As time goes by, the paradigm may continue to stand but now a little rickety, wounded, supported by intellectual crutches. It is an interesting phenomenon of the human mind that it requires some model—no matter how bad—to explain a natural phenomenon, and the old model will not be abandoned until there is something to replace it. The intellect hates vacuums.

In time, someone presents a new model, one compatible with the data that assailed the old, and the scientist-usurpers put forward their challenge to the king/queen on his/her paradigmatic throne. Thereupon the field enters a period of crisis, or even chaos. There is much coming and going: the defenders of the Old Faith rally to the support of the model learned from their revered mentors, but the revolutionaries continue to attack the gates, now splintered and weak. During this period scientific controversy thrives. Letters are written to the editors of scientific periodicals; harsh words are said in public and in private. The turmoil may even erode personal relations, for often reputations, success, and recognition are associated with the perceived validity of a model. If the model goes, then the status of its adherents may be under attack or even wiped out, cast away, and trashed. Gradually, as more data accumulate, the new paradigm gets more and more support from the cognoscenti and becomes enthroned as the prevailing and accepted ideal. And now it is the turn of the new paradigm to attract experimental attack, until it too follows the path of its predecessor to rejection and replacement.

Irrespective of its impact on scientific thought, Kuhn's thesis was useful to us for its explanation of the psychological reaction of our colleagues. We now realized that we had replaced a previously existing paradigm and were passing through the period of "crisis," with its expected attendant furor, before a new paradigm—that is, our claim to have identified the hepatitis virus—was accepted. This knowledge had a calming effect on us, for, according to Kuhn, the fuss would soon pass if our model continued to withstand the onslaught of experimental testing and became the new paradigm.

On one occasion, a colleague, Dr. William Summerskill, a distinguished liver physician from the Mayo Clinic, told Alton Sutnick that the longtime workers in the field were annoyed that our work had suddenly appeared, making claims for the discovery of the virus they had sought for so many years. Al's response was, "You'll get over it." And they eventually did.

We are not the only scientists to derive clarity and comfort from Kuhn's analysis of the social context of revolutionary scientific change. In 1977, Carl Woese, an evolutionary microbiologist at the University of Illinois, announced the discovery of the archaea, one-celled organisms that were very different from all other living things, including the bacteria with which they had previously been classified. Henceforth, he claimed, instead of two domains of life, prokaryotes (without a nucleus) and eukaryotes (with a nucleus), there were now three: bacteria, archaea (mostly unicellular organisms), and eucarya (multicellular organisms). There were many doubters, and it took years before the importance and validity of his contribution was recognized. The clincher, both scientifically and psychologically, came in 1996 when the complete genetic sequence of one of the archaea, *Methanococcus jannaschi*, was published. It had a large number of genes not found in other domains and was more similar to the eucarya than to the bacteria. Amazingly, the organisms shared about one-third of their genes with mammals! The shared sequences had been conserved in contemporary "higher" forms since the origins of cellular life. Woese, when he was interviewed for *Science* magazine in 1998,[23] said, in reference to his deferred recognition:

> That's what happens when you break a paradigm; people scoff, they don't treat you seriously. But I'd read Thomas Kuhn, so I knew exactly what was going on.

Kuhn's views have had great play in the field of philosophy of science. They have been interpreted to mean that science is a socially driven activity without the guidance of logic and reason; they have been contrasted with the Popperian rigor of hypothesis rejection. These debates, which at times distort Kuhn's views, seem to me to be of limited value. What I know is that his insights were of great help to others and to us.

[23] V. Morell, "Microbiology's Scarred Revolutionary," *Science* 276 (1998): 699–702.

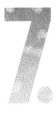

Identifying the Hepatitis B Virus

By 1967 we had established and published a report[1] on the association between the Australia antigen and patients with hepatitis. But the association, although highly significant statistically and supported in several studies in our laboratory and elsewhere, was not proof enough that the quaintly named Australia antigen could be equated with hepatitis virus. We had to show that it had other characteristics of a virus and a causal relation to the disease. It is embarrassing to admit, but at the time I was woefully ignorant about viruses. Virology was not a big-ticket item in the medical school curriculum in the late 1940s, and there was remarkably little knowledge of or treatment for viruses in the clinical experience I had during my medical and surgical hospital training. Nor had my colleagues had a much richer experience than I. So we went to the bookshelf, took down the volume marked "Virology," and looked up the characteristics of a virus.

    1. *Viruses can be visualized as regular-shaped particles in the electron microscope. The expected size range of hepatitis virus was known from filtration experiments that had been done prior to our work.*

    2. *Viruses contain nucleic acid, either DNA or RNA, that is required for the replication process.*

    3. *Viruses can often be grown in tissue or organ cultures.*

[1] B. S. Blumberg, B.J.S. Gerstley, D. A. Hungerford, W. T. London, and A. I. Sutnick, "A Serum Antigen (Australia Antigen) in Down's Syndrome Leukemia and Hepatitis," *Annals of Internal Medicine* 66 (1967): 924–31.

4. *Some viruses form plaques in thinly spread cells that are susceptible to the virus.*[2]

5. *There was the expectation that the putative virus, which we postulated was in the fraction of the blood that contained Australia antigen, would fulfill Koch's postulates. We will get to this after I discuss the first points.*

We followed the duck strategy: that is, if something walks like a duck, quacks like a duck, swims like a duck, flies like a duck, and so forth, then it is more likely to be a duck than, let's say, a great blue heron. It is a trivial designation for a very powerful scientific method, namely, the concept of independent evidence.

There is a method widely used among virologists for isolating viruses from biological materials, such as blood. The fluid is placed in a tube with a material such as sugar solution that increases its density. The tube is spun in an ultracentrifuge, which places an extremely high gravitational pull on the molecules in the fluid, including the virus. The protein particles and the viruses will move to a place in the tube that reflects their molecular weight. Then, drops of the fluid are collected in separate containers as they emerge from a pinhole in the bottom of the centrifuge tube where the molecules have layered according to their molecular weight. A test is done on each of the collection tubes to determine which fraction (or fractions) contain(s) the hypothesized virus. In our study we used the immunodiffusion test for the surface antigen of HBV, which has already been described, and identified the tubes containing what we thought might be the hepatitis virus.

There was a powerful electron microscope (EM) group at Fox Chase Cancer Center. Thomas Anderson, its director, had been one of the first scientists in America to use the EM on biological material and was probably the first to visualize a phage—that is, a virus that

---

[2] The plaque assay was one of the first techniques used for detecting and isolating viruses. Its first use, probably, was in 1915 when Félix d'Hérelle noted that viruses that infect bacteria—bacteriophages—will kill the bacteria they invade and leave a hole or plaque in the lawn of bacteria spread on an agar plate. It was later found that layers of other cells from humans and other animals could also be used to show the presence of the virus and, under some circumstances, to isolate it.

infects bacteria—an important step in the development of molecular biology.[3] Working with him was Manfred Bayer, who had considerable experience looking at the cell walls of bacteria and also modeling the appearance of the phage virus. Barbara Werner[4] helped to isolate the virus, and we provided a small amount of it to Manfred. Within a short time we were called to see what he had found.

Manfred is a painstaking scientist with a meticulous approach to the craft of microscopy. It took him some time to select the correct shadowing methods for the preparations and to decide exactly where to look. In the ultracentrifuge fraction that contained the Australia antigen, he saw particles that were roughly circular, about 210 angstroms[5] in diameter, and whose centers were, for the most part, empty. The particles were pretty small for a virus, but, as we concluded in the published paper,[6] they could be the sought-after hepatitis B virus.

---

[3] Horace Freeland Judson, in his monumental history of the origins of molecular biology (*The Eighth Day of Creation* [New York: Simon and Schuster, 1979]), provides an excellent description of Anderson's significant contribution to molecular biology. Judson quotes Anderson: "We could really see the phage as tadpole-shaped particles, whose heads ranged from 600 to 800 A in diameter, depending on the species. . . . There was no doubt in our minds that we had found the phage particles, but certain other workers remained skeptical for years. . . . I remember particularly the reaction of Alfred Hershey's teacher, kindly old Professor J. J. Bronfenbrenner, who had worked on bacteriophages for many years at Washington University in St. Louis. When he first saw our pictures he clapped the palm of his hand to his forehead and exclaimed, '*Mein Gott!* They've got tails!'"

In addition to his excellent accounts of science, Judson has achieved a niche in the annals of Bob Dylan fandom. He is the harassed journalist interviewing Bob in the 1967 cult film *Don't Look Back*, which depicts Dylan's tour of Great Britain in 1965.

[4] Barbara has the distinction of having diagnosed what was probably the first case of clinical hepatitis detected serologically—her own! In the spring of 1967, she developed symptoms of hepatitis, tested her serum, and found Australia antigen. She went on to full recovery. Her timely use of the serological test reinforced our belief that Au was associated with hepatitis.

[5] The angstrom unit is named after Anders J. Ångström (1814–74), a Swedish physicist. It is equal to 10^{-8}cm—that is, one one-hundred-millionth of a centimeter.

[6] M. E. Bayer, B. S. Blumberg, and B. Werner, "Particles Associated with Australia Antigen in the Sera of Patients with Leukemia, Down's Syndrome and Hepatitis," *Nature* 218 (1968): 1057–59.

Did it contain nucleic acid, which would be expected if it was a virus? Irv Millman, with his amazing capacity to learn and develop laboratory skills as they were needed, and another of our colleagues at Fox Chase, Lawrence Loeb (later, professor of pathology at the University of Washington in Seattle), studied the physical and other characteristics of the particles. They did not contain nucleic acid, at least within the sensitivity of the tests we used. We postulated, in 1969, that other particles we had not yet observed were the whole virus, and that the particles we had seen were associated with the virus. It wasn't until 1970 that a group of British scientists led by Dr. D. S. Dane reported visualizing the whole virus particle that did include nucleic acid.[7]

In the interim period, before the nucleic acid–containing virus was identified and verified, we had wild ideas that we had found a new class of infectious agents that could produce protein from protein without the presence of nucleic acid. This was highly speculative, since it would have shattered an arm of the so-called central dogma advanced by Francis Crick, the codiscoverer (along with James Watson) of the structure of DNA. The "dogma" postulated a unidirectional vector from DNA that produced RNA, which then produced protein. A part of the dogma was exploded when the (1975) Nobel Prize winners David Baltimore, Renato Dulbecco, and Howard Temin showed that in some viruses RNA can produce DNA by the use of an enzyme called reverse transcriptase.

I am a determined (and ordinarily frustrated) neologist—a maker of new words—and this concept cried out for word-creative action. We termed the agents associated with Australia antigen "ICRONS." This was an acronym merging the initials of the Institute for Cancer Research with the terminal Greek suffix "on,"[8] with its vague reference to particle-like entities (cf. ion, proton, electron, etc.). Ironically (nearly a good pun), at about this time Carleton Gajdusek was beginning to formulate his ideas about an infectious agent that caused

[7] D. S. Dane, C. H. Cameron, and M. Briggs, "Virus-like Particles in the Serum of Patients with Australia Antigen Associated Hepatitis," *Lancet* 1 (1970): 695.

[8] The suffix "-on" derives from the Ionians, ancient inhabitants of the Peloponnese who mysteriously entered ancient Greece as wanderers. This gave an additional symbolic character to the word.

the strange neurological disease kuru, found among the Fore people of Papua New Guinea. He postulated that it might be an agent composed only of protein, and that it was spread by cannibalism. This, in due course, resulted in the discovery of the strange "prion" agents[9] that do not appear to have nucleic acid. If this model continues to be supported and a nucleic acid–containing particle is not found, another element of the dogma will be changed. So much for scientific dogmas.[10]

We tried very hard to grow the putative virus in tissue or organ culture. Scott Mazzur had joined us in January of 1969 after she had completed several years of training in the laboratory of the noted virologists Werner and Gertrude Henle. Scott tried, for three years, to develop an effective tissue or organ culture in which to grow the virus. But despite her excellent training and experience, she was unsuccessful. Scott changed direction and made very important discoveries concerning the subtypes of HBV. Even now, when we know so much more than we did in the early days, it has not been possible to grow HBV in conventional tissue cultures. Nor, for technical reasons we did not fully unravel, were the plaque assays feasible. At this point we were partly satisfied that we had identified a fraction containing a virus, but more support for the hypothesis was needed, and so we turned to the traditional Koch postulates.

Robert Koch (1843–1910)[11] and others have stated the postulates in various formats, and modern techniques and knowledge have modified them considerably. We used the following articulation.

- *The suspected agent is associated with the disease in question. In some formulations it is found in* all *cases of the disease.*

[9] For which, in 1997, Stanley B. Prusiner was awarded the Nobel Prize.

[10] Professor Crick had been criticized for using the term "dogma," borrowed from religion, for a scientific model. "Dogma" implies that the concept is accepted without proof, resting on the power of authority. Crick claimed that he used the term in an entirely different sense, applying it to an idea that was without proof and therefore without powerful standing.

[11] Robert Koch was among the early pioneers, including Louis Pasteur, Edwin Klebs, Ferdinand Cohn, and others, who established the germ theory of disease. Koch's mentor, Friedrich Gustav Jacob Henle, contributed significantly to the postulates, which are therefore sometimes referred to as the "Henle-Koch Postulates."

- *The suspected agent is removed from the affected tissues of a patient with the disease and grown in pure culture outside the original host. Viruses require cells and tissues to grow in rather than the cell-free media that can nourish bacteria.*
- *The isolated suspected agent is then transmitted to an experimental animal.*
- *The infected animals develop the same disease as the patient.*
- *The suspected agent is then isolated from the infected animal and transmitted to a second experimental animal.*
- *The second animal develops the same disease as the patient.*

How could we satisfy the postulates and add evidence to our hypothesis that we had indeed discovered a hepatitis virus? The candidate viral material—Australia antigen—had been found in the blood and liver of many patients with hepatitis, thus supporting the first postulate. We had observed that donor blood containing Au could transmit Au to the recipient of these bloods. (The practice of using donor bloods containing Au was terminated after we knew that we could routinely identify Au in donor blood.) This in a way satisfied, by analogy, the second postulate. However, in order to more fully confirm the hypothesis of infectious transmission, and from this be able to go on to the application of the research to the saving of human lives, we needed additional confirmation. A few carefully designed animal studies would be required. First, we had to determine which species of animals could be used for the testing. On the basis of a large series of observations we identified a few species, including several nonhuman primates, that could become "naturally" infected with the putative virus. (The primates that had been infected did not appear to have any symptoms due to the infection.) This process greatly decreased the number of animals we would have to use.

In the 1960s and 1970s, the National Cancer Institute was conducting extensive studies on the viral cause of cancer, an important part of the research campaign to control the growing cancer morbidity and mortality. They used vervet monkeys (family *Cercopithecus*) specifically raised for the project. Through the courtesy of the director, we were allowed to use several of these, and Tom London played the major role in the subsequent studies. Material containing Australia antigen was inoculated into the monkeys, and they were observed for a few weeks. Several developed Australia antigen after the inoculation. In one case, Tom took blood from the infected vervet in which the Australia antigen had apparently replicated and then inoculated it into a second vervet. The second animal also developed the Australia antigen; we had fulfilled another of the Koch postulates. These animal experiments, although small in number, were very important in moving the research forward.

We were doing pretty well on the postulates, if all the observations and experiments were considered together. True, they had not been satisfied exactly—for example, the experimental animals did not develop clinical hepatitis—but, taken along with our other studies, these findings began to sound pretty convincing. Science may not always bring us to the truth, but it does tell us when to get on to the next step, including application.

In October of 1968 we began to distribute—gratis, to scientists who requested them—reagent kits consisting of a serum containing Australia antigen and a second serum containing the antibody against it (anti-HBs). This was one of the best steps we could have taken to move the research forward and speed its application. For years afterward, I met scientists in many parts of the world who recalled how these reagents allowed them to start research immediately without spending a year or more trying to find the reagents by themselves.

Tom London and Irv Millman made another unexpected observation that, in retrospect, had a major bearing on what is probably the most important practical outcome of all our research—that is, the invention of the hepatitis B vaccine. They found that when the highly purified fraction of Australia antigen was used in the injection experiments, infection did not occur. But if a less purified material was used, the vervet became infected. We also knew that the Australia antigen particles appeared to be hollow, and that the purified fractions did not contain nucleic acid. From this we could infer that the purification process had separated the infectious particle that pre-

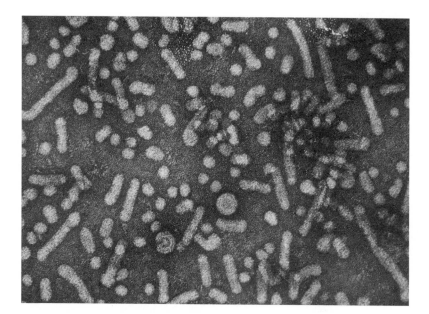

Fig. 2. An electron micrograph of the HBV particles, showing the large, small, and elongated particles.

sumably could cause disease—and which we had not yet seen—from the noninfectious particles that we had observed in the EM.

During the next few months and years a growing understanding of the virus emerged. Some of this work was done at Fox Chase Cancer Center, but most of it was accomplished in laboratories spread throughout the world. A large number of investigators entered the field, and research on hepatitis became a minor growth industry. It was said, facetiously (this was before the connection between chronic liver disease and cancer of the liver was fully realized), that more people had made a living from HBV than had died from it. I once received a telegram from a group of clinical laboratory workers who were employed to test donor blood for HBV, thanking me for their jobs!

The virus, HBV (figs. 2 and 3) is about forty-two nanometers (a nanometer is one-billionth of a meter) in diameter, one of the smallest DNA viruses that infect humans. The surface antigen—that is,

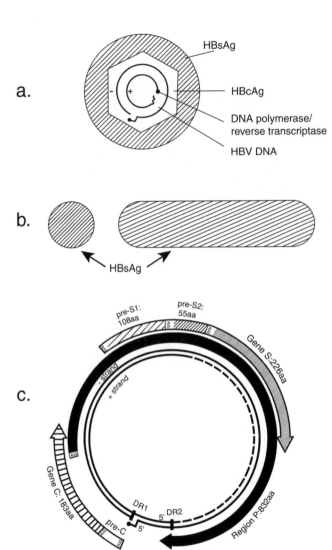

Fig. 3. (a) The structure of the hepatitis B virus, showing the surface antigen (HBsAg) that surrounds the whole virus and the core antigen (HbcAg) that surrounds the circular DNA strands. The strands are double, with a large gap in the inner (positive) strand. The outer (negative) strand is complete. The DNA polymerase acts on the DNA strand. The overall size of the virus is forty-two nanometers. **(b)** The smaller particles that contain only HBsAg. The circular particle is twenty-four nanometers in diameter, and the elongated particles are the same diameter but of variable length. **(c)** The DNA viral genome of HBV, showing the complete outer strand and the inner strand with the gap indicated. The location of the four open reading frames, *S, C, P,* and *X*, are shown along with the number of amino acids they contain. They are described in greater detail in Appendix 4.

the protein that forms an envelope around the outside of the virus—was designated hepatitis B surface antigen (HBsAg); this was a new name for what we had called Australia antigen. The strands of DNA that make up the viral genes are nestled inside the virus and are surrounded by the core antigen (HBcAg). The length of the viral DNA—its genome—is about thirty-two hundred units (base pairs), one of the smallest genomes of any human virus.[12] This provides for only four genes that could produce a few proteins of moderate or small size. HBV is about as simple as viruses can get, at least in its biochemical and physical equipment. Its "behavior," as we shall see, is far from simple.

In addition to the whole virus particle I have just described, there are two other kinds of particles that are made entirely of the surface antigen (HBsAg) without any DNA or genes in them (fig. 2). These particles are not infectious, and they cannot multiply or directly cause disease. One is a roughly circular particle about twenty-two nanometers in diameter; this is the particle that we saw in the first electron microscope pictures. There are, in addition, elongated particles of the same diameter as the spherical ones, but of varying lengths. There are many more of the noninfectious HBsAg particles (without DNA) in the blood than whole virus particles that are infectious and can replicate; in natural infections the ratio is about 1000:1. It is this feature of the virus that made possible the invention of the unique vaccine for HBV. In a later chapter, I will discuss the molecular biology of HBV that has emerged in the research of the past few years. Oddly, most of the important applications of the research on HBV were realized before there was a significant understanding of the virus's molecular details.

When the surface antigen (HBsAg) is detected in the blood—this was originally done by the immunodiffusion method and later by the much more sensitive radioimmunoassay and enzyme-based

---

[12] Hepatitis D virus (HDV)—an RNA virus—has a smaller genome, about seventeen hundred base pairs. It cannot infect people unless they are previously infected with HBV or there is a coinfection. HDV is "clothed" in HBsAg, although it has a different mix of the basic proteins that make up HBsAg from HBV.

assays—it indicates the presence of either the whole virus, or the smaller particles that contain only HBsAg and no DNA, or both. The first antibody that we found, the antibody present in the hemophilia patient from New York, was directed against HBsAg and, in the standard nomenclature, is referred to as anti-HBs. There is also an antibody against the core antigen, and it is designated anti-HBc. There is another protein related to the HBcAg, designated as HBeAg, whose presence indicates active replication of the virus. When the antibody against this protein, anti-HBe, is found in the blood, it is usually an indication that replication has diminished or stopped.

In the mid-1970s and later the pattern of serological and clinical responses to HBV infection was established. There are several outcomes following infection. Most infected people will develop anti-HBs without any evidence of disease and retain lifelong protection against further infection. A second group will develop acute hepatitis, which may last for weeks or months, followed in most cases by complete recovery and, again, lifelong protection. About 5 percent of patients with acute hepatitis will develop chronic infection, and this can, in some of the cases, lead to liver failure, premature death, and/or cancer of the liver. About 1 percent of patients with acute hepatitis develop a rapid and usually deadly form of the disease—fulminant hepatitis—for which treatment is very difficult. From 0.1 percent to over 20 percent of those infected—depending on the geographic location and other characteristics of the population—will become HBV *carriers*. They do not develop acute disease or anti-HBs but retain the virus and become chronically infected with HBV, and HBsAg can be detected in their blood. The term "carrier" is usually defined to mean an individual who has the virus in his or her blood, liver, or other tissue but has no subjective evidence of disease, that is, no symptoms. Carriers may remain infected, but asymptomatic, for years. They are, however, at risk for chronic liver disease that can lead to failure of liver function. They are also at greatly increased risk for primary cancer of the liver, a deadly and difficult-to-treat illness. The serological and clinical course of acute and chronic disease is shown in figure 4.

Acute Hepatitis B

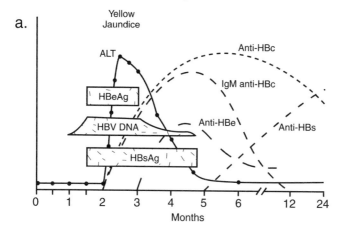

Chronic Hepatitis B

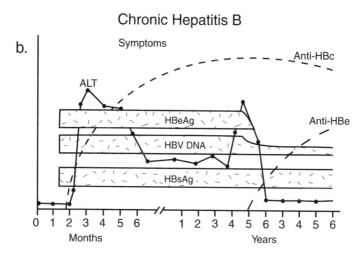

Fig. 4. Serological patterns during the course of acute (top) and chronic (bottom) hepatitis B infection. The times of appearance and (sometimes) disappearance of various markers for "typical" cases are shown. ALT is an enzyme that appears in the blood and reflects the extent of liver damage. In the acute case, the surface antigen, HBsAg, the HBV DNA, and the HbeAg (derived from the *C* reading frame) appear early in the course of the disease and then decrease or disappear. In the chronic case, they persist for months and years. In the acute case, the antibodies against various components, anti-HBc, anti-HBe, and anti-HBs, appear at different times. (Anti-HBc comes in two forms, which are carried in different fractions of the immune gamma globulin [Ig]. There is an earlier IgM anti-HBc and a later anti-HBc carried in the IgG fraction.) The antibody pattern in the chronic cases is quite different and often does not include the protective anti-HBs. (Adapted from *IARC Monographs on the Evaluation of Carcinogenic Risks to Humans*, vol. 59, *Hepatitis Viruses* [Lyons: IARC, 1994], 60.)

We had passed through a period of intense research and discovery, and we and the other scientists and physicians in the field were beginning to appreciate how the infection started and advanced. These discoveries had emerged from our interest in the basic science of disease susceptibility and resistance. The thrill of discovery and science for its own sake are attractive parts of the scientific endeavor, but we were now ready to help apply our discoveries to matters of life and death.

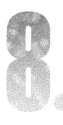
The Control of Posttransfusion Hepatitis

By 1967 we were ready to apply our research to practical medical needs. The test for Australia antigen could be used to detect hepatitis in occult carriers and to diagnose patients with hepatitis B. Although the tests were insensitive and there was ample scope for improvement, it appeared that they would be useful. The lesson of life is that the solution of one problem usually raises others, and medicine is not exempt from this dictum. The events of the next few years provided good examples of this truism with regard to HBV.

In the 1960s, the blood collection and transfusion "industry" in the United States was growing rapidly. Although a sizable percentage of the blood was collected by not-for-profit organizations, primarily the American Red Cross and hospital blood banks, for-profit companies were collecting a significant part of it. An individual or company could set up a "blood bank," buy blood at low cost from "professional" donors, and then sell it to hospitals and physicians at a significant multiple of the acquisition price. These enterprises flourished because of the explosive growth of surgery after World War II. Improvements in anesthesia and the availability of antibiotics to combat pre- and postoperative infections allowed—in fact, encouraged—much longer and more ambitious surgical procedures. For example, open-heart surgery to treat diseased heart valves and congenital defects, radical cancer surgery, and renal transplantation were significantly more widely practiced by the 1960s than they had been before.

These important medical advances created problems. Longer and more demanding procedures required large numbers of blood transfusions, and posttransfusion hepatitis was widespread. In some of the studies done in the centers where these "heroic" surgical procedures were common, as many as 50 percent of the patients who received multiple transfusions developed hepatitis weeks or months after the surgery. Although these attacks were only occasionally fatal, it was not pleasant for a patient to suffer the misery of a protracted period of jaundice and the other nasty symptoms that accompany hepatitis infection while trying to recover from major surgery.

Before our discovery of Australia antigen there was no method to detect hepatitis in the blood of infectious donors and remove the contaminated units from the blood supply. As we continued to amass evidence that the Australia antigen identified parts of the hepatitis B virus, we realized that we could use the immunodiffusion test to detect asymptomatic carriers. Many blood bank scientists were not aware of our claim that we had identified a hepatitis virus, and among those who were, there was the natural skepticism concerning any new idea that upset an established model. Although we could infer from the evidence that it was likely that we had detected the virus, there was no direct scientific evidence that we could decrease the incidence of posttransfusion hepatitis by testing and removing the positive units. We were told that the medical and blood-banking community would not change their practices based on the available evidence. In addition to the changes required in their day-to-day operations, there would be increased costs that could cut into profits for the entrepreneurial blood bank supplier and impact the economies of the not-for-profit health institutions. We needed to plan a research project that would compel the blood-banking community to take notice.

We designed an elaborate study to test the hypothesis that removing the donor blood units that contained Australia antigen from the donor pool would decrease the incidence of posttransfusion hepatitis. Tom London, Alton Sutnick, and I were, at the time, attending physicians at several hospitals in Philadelphia. One of these was Philadelphia General Hospital, a large city-owned institution in West Philadelphia adjacent to the Medical School of the University of Pennsylvania, which it served as a teaching facility. It was an ancient establishment first opened as an almshouse in 1732. (It was active during the Civil War; my wife Jean's great-grandfather, Maurice Weinstein, a sergeant in the Sixty-sixth Regiment, New York Infantry, was probably a patient there in the summer of 1862.) Though often crowded and beset with many of the problems of a large urban public institution, it was well staffed and had a strong tradition of clinical research. John Senior, one of the university physicians on service at PGH, had long and extensive experience with hepatitis. He had studied the incidence of posttransfusion hepatitis at PGH over the course of several years and knew that it was high, and probably higher than at other institutions in the city. For our study, the activities of the blood bank would continue as they had before, but we would be given a sample of the donor blood to test for Australia antigen.[1] Patients who had received a "positive" unit would be followed regularly during their hospital stay and during their convalescence at home, and data would be collected on the incidence of hepatitis events (i.e., clinical symptoms and signs of hepatitis, and/or changes in the serology that signaled infection). At the same time a control patient would be identified who had received a unit that was not positive, and he or she would also be followed. After a sufficient number of patients had been enrolled and followed, we could determine whether the incidence of hepatitis events was more common in those who had received the positive units than in those who had received negative units. Remember, although we *suspected* that we had identified the agent that caused posttransfusion hepatitis, we did not have evidence to convince others that this was the case. The research project was essential to determine how we should proceed.

The research plan was submitted to the Clinical Investigation Review Committee at Fox Chase Cancer Center. They approved the plan and encouraged us to move ahead with appropriate speed to

[1] In routine blood bank practice at the time, when blood was taken to fill the donor unit container, a small sample was placed in a "pilot tube," to be used for red cell antigen testing and cross-matching to ensure that the donor and patient were compatible. A small amount of this blood was used for the Australia antigen test, so there was no additional inconvenience to the patient.

allow application as soon as possible, if the results supported the hypothesis. The study commenced late in 1968 (about a year after the publication of our first paper hypothesizing that Australia antigen was part of a hepatitis virus), and the slow accumulation of data began. On 26 June 26 1969 my friend and colleague Dr. Kazuo Okochi, then at the Blood Bank of the University of Tokyo, came to visit FCCC. We had previously met during my first field trip to Japan in September of 1965. We shared an interest in iso-antibodies against serum proteins, and Kazuo had been a contributor to the research on the lipoprotein polymorphism. During my 1965 visit to Japan I had spoken about Australia antigen, although at the time the association with hepatitis was only suspected. Later, Kazuo had identified an antibody against Australia antigen and sent it to me for comparison with the antisera we had identified. He was also one of the first to confirm the association between hepatitis and Australia antigen.

Kazuo had some interesting news for us. He had begun testing, in Tokyo, the same hypothesis we were testing at Philadelphia General Hospital. He had proceeded more rapidly than we had, and his results were already significant. There were several reasons he moved faster than we did. Carriers of HBV, Australia antigen–positive donors, were much more common in Japan than in the United States. In our first surveys, we had found a prevalence of about 0.1 percent in the United States, while in Japan it was five to ten times greater. The higher prevalence meant that the carriers could be found several times more rapidly than in our study. In addition, in Japan the donor units were smaller than in the United States, and it was more likely that a Japanese patient would receive transfusions from a larger number of people. Whatever the reasons, the numbers in his study were already large enough to achieve statistical significance, and he was able to state that the hypothesis had been supported.

Kazuo's impressive finding required—to use the cliché of the time—an agonizing reappraisal of our strategy. Prior to viewing Kazuo's data, we were ethically obligated to test the hypothesis. If we did not, the procedure might not be accepted, or its acceptance would be long delayed. Should we now accept the hypothesis as adequately supported by Kazuo's data? Was it now ethical to stop the experiment and adopt the procedure as standard medical practice? The number of patients Kazuo had studied was not large: 19 of 58 patients who had received at least one unit of blood with Au(+) blood (i.e., blood that tested positive for Australia antigen) became Au(+) 15 to 110 days after transfusion, while only 10 of 99 patients who received Au(-) blood did so.[2] However, the difference was statistically significant.

Ultimately, we did decide that the hypothesis had been adequately tested; we had great confidence in Kazuo, and the data pointed in the same direction as did our early results at Philadelphia General Hospital. Further, the conviction that Au was part of the virus was growing stronger day by day, and all this added to the logic that we could prevent disease. We stopped the experiment, but we did not stop testing the blood. Beginning in July 1969, it was no longer an experiment but an applied hospital routine. We maintained the program for the Philadelphia General Hospital until commercial testing resources became available. Several years later, John Senior, his colleagues, and we published a paper that compared the incidence of posttransfusion hepatitis before and after the institution of routine testing. In the 1968–69 period, before testing, it was 18 percent. In the 1970–71 period, after testing had been in place for about a year, the incidence was 6 percent, a decrease of about two-thirds—a formidable, although by no means perfect, outcome. However, in medicine we rarely have perfect results; early methods usually improve incrementally with time and further research.

When does research end and application begin?—this is a question that often arises in the practice of medicine. We could nearly pinpoint the day—late June to early July 1969—when our research project at Philadelphia General Hospital was applied. Our decision to use the test as a standard medical procedure determined its destiny—if we were doing it, then other blood banks and hospitals had to decide why they should not do so.

The fact that we were convinced did not mean that others were. In 1969 Tom London, Alton Sutnick, and I had written a short paper

---

[2] Okochi later published his results, first in 1968 (*Vox Sang* 15 [1968]: 374) and more fully in 1970.

in the *Bulletin of Pathology*[3]—not a journal of wide distribution but one that was likely to be seen by many in the blood-banking and clinical laboratory world—in which we suggested that the "Au test" should be used for screening blood donors, and that we were doing so in Philadelphia. This did not elicit a major response, as far as I could tell. I did receive a request from a colleague in the blood-banking fraternity that I retract the article. He opined that it was premature, and that the conclusion was based on insufficient evidence. His was a tenable position: the data were not massive, and it was a value judgment as to whether they were sufficient. However, events soon swept away any equivocation.

What happened between our initial testing and the the screening procedure's acceptance by the medical community? Our early data from the Philadelphia General Hospital study became available, and D. J. Gocke and N. B. Kavey in New Jersey published another small series that was similar to Kazuo's findings, but there wasn't much more than that. Our findings and those of the others prompted a review by an expert panel of the Division of Medical Sciences of the National Research Council.[4] At a meeting convened at the National Academy of Sciences on 31 October and 1 November 1969, they recommended that the results of the studies on Australia antigen be reviewed, and that a routinely applicable test be developed on the basis of those that had been used in the research projects. They did not recommend immediate certification of the available test, because they estimated that it detected only about 25 percent of the HBV carriers and hepatitis cases. Others, however, were more impressed with the data.

In July of 1970 Harvey Alter (the selfsame Harvey who had been the first to see the Australia antigen precipitin band in our laboratory and was now on the staff of the Blood Bank at the National

---

[3] B. S. Blumberg, W. T. London, and A. I. Sutnick, "Relation of Australia Antigen to Virus of Hepatitis," *Bulletin of Pathology* 10 (1969): 164.

[4] The National Research Council is the operating arm of the National Academy of Sciences. They help to fulfill the function assigned to the NAS of responding to scientific questions posed by the federal government. They also may generate projects on their own initiative.

Institutes of Health), Paul Schmidt,[5] the director of the NIH Blood Bank and a scientific and professional leader in the field, and Paul Holland, also at the Blood Bank, forcefully entered the scene. On the basis of essentially the same data that were available to the NRC committee, they recommended that all blood banks capable of testing for Au should do so, despite the low sensitivity. They wrote:

> [T]he actual incidence of post-transfusion hepatitis in the United States exceeds 150,000 cases a year. Granted that, with current detection techniques, the exclusion of HAA-positive [i.e., Au(+)] donors would prevent no more than 25% of these cases, this still represents a highly significant decrease in hepatitis-related morbidity and mortality. The National Research Council has viewed this 25% detection-rate as representing an inability to prevent 75% of the cases of post-transfusion hepatitis. Ruling out 25% of potentially infectious blood-donors and preventing 40,000 cases of hepatitis a year is a more positive and useful approach.[6]

There was no reason to allow the perfect to drive out the good. Again, it is a lesson learned from evolution: nature evolves to "getting by," not perfection. On 29 July 29 1970 the *New York Times* reported (on a back page)[7] the findings from the NIH blood bank scientists and their strong recommendation that testing be started.

After that, things began to move; the pace of life quickened. The Alter article led to a reconvening of the NRC committee on 5 October 1970, and they changed their recommendation to encourage testing in laboratories that were able to do so. They prepared their report very rapidly, and at the meeting of the American Association

[5] I am indebted to Dr. Schmidt, then at the Southwest Florida Blood Bank in Tampa, Florida, who, in a letter of 26 September 1997, provided me with the chronology of events concerning blood testing.

[6] *Lancet* 2 (July 1970): 142.

[7] The media never developed much of an interest in hepatitis. "Popular" infectious agents (in particular, HIV) were often front-page news and the subject of the evening newscasts, generating opinions, comments, and talk show phone-ins. HBV had a much more modest lifestyle, and workers in the field plodded along with their various successes, for the most part unheralded and unheeded. There were advantages to working in relative obscurity, but the downside was that there was less public financial support.

of Blood Banks in San Francisco on 29 October it was presented by Dr. James Sgouris at a session on hepatitis chaired by Paul Schmidt. At the same meeting Dr. James M. Stengle of the National Heart and Lung Institute announced that they would be prepared to send reagents to laboratories and blood banks that requested them. This allowed us to stop our program of reagent distribution, although my recollection is that we continued to send reagents to foreign laboratories that might have had difficulty using the U.S. government resources. Therefore, October 1970 can be taken as the date when the use of the test became "official." This was followed by a series of laws and regulations. In 1971, the New York state legislature passed a law requiring testing. In June 1972 the American Association of Blood Banks, in their book of standards, required the testing of donors. In July 1972 the *Federal Register* published the requirement for testing of all blood used in interstate commerce, and the following year it was required of all blood banks. I was against the passing of legislation, preferring the use of health department regulation to define the acceptable procedure. It is very difficult to frame medical goals in the legal terminology required for legislation. Furthermore, it is difficult to change the law in the face of new findings, which always emerge in a scientific program that is constantly seeking innovation. Departmental rules are easier to modify.

In addition to the legislation and health regulations, litigation, I suspect, became a strong motivation for the initiation of testing. Beginning in 1969, we became aware that legal action was being taken against blood banks, hospitals, and physicians by patients (and their families) who had contracted posttransfusion hepatitis. In part, the claims of the plaintiffs were based on the failure of the blood banks to test for Australia antigen. Suddenly, there was an increase in requests to us for the reagents needed for testing. The threat of a painful malpractice suit can, apparently, focus the mind more effectively than rational scientific argument. Although physicians are often bitter about the effects of malpractice suits, it is possible that, in this instance, the specter of such litigation accelerated the application of donor testing.

By the mid-1970s, posttransfusion hepatitis due to HBV had essentially disappeared from the United States and the other countries where compulsory testing had been instituted. The lives preserved, the illnesses prevented, the reclamation of productive work time, the hundreds of millions of dollars saved on medical care—all this repaid manyfold the money that society had invested in our research and that of our colleagues. What had started out as an esoteric investigation of human diversity in America, Africa, Asia, and the Pacific resulted in a significant medical advance and, as the politicians now refer to it, "wealth generation" for the pharmaceutical and diagnostic companies, their shareholders, and the new employees required for this advancement in the medical business.

Solving One Problem Creates Others

Perfect solutions are not often within the grasp of questing humanity. How often do we have the experience in our everyday life that the solution of one problem seems, after an appropriate period of celebration, to reveal others? So it is with the scientific process.

A good advance was achieved when the methods for the detection of HBsAg were greatly improved, first by the introduction of the radioimmunoassay and by later enzyme-based assays. These were many times more sensitive than the immunodiffusion method we had introduced. But even with these advances, there were still cases of posttransfusion hepatitis, and it became apparent that there was at least one other blood-borne virus that caused hepatitis. In the mid-1980s hepatitis C virus (HCV) was discovered, and a method for testing donor blood became available. With the use of these two tests—HBV and HCV—posttransfusion hepatitis became even more rare; for the present, it is under reasonably good control. Other hepatitis viruses have been discovered—D, E, and G—and probably additional ones will be found in the future. At least one of these, and probably more, can be transmitted by transfusion, but they do not appear to be as much of a clinical problem as B and C have been in the past. Ongoing vigilance is the marching cry of preventive medicine.

There was another problem that arose as a consequence of the testing. Beginning about 1968, when testing for Au had started in Philadelphia, we began to hear reports of people, mostly healthcare workers, who had been disadvantaged as a consequence of their identification as hepatitis carriers. For example, a hospital nurse was found to be a carrier. She was told that she would be fired because she might infect others, and the hospital was fearful of malpractice suits that might result from her activities. An applicant for a hospital position was deemed unacceptable because he was a carrier. A homosexual young man who was employed in a health-care clinic was informed that he was a carrier, and that he would have to leave his position. Moreover, he and the other carriers were not told how they should conduct themselves socially. With the mainstreaming of many mentally retarded children, some carriers were introduced into classrooms in the absence of any knowledge as to which children were carriers or what precautions should be taken. The discovery of a carrier child in a classroom would raise fear in the parents of the other children and, in some cases, ostracism of the infected child.

A particularly dramatic problem arose with respect to renal dialysis clinics. There were many reports in the United States and elsewhere in the world of hepatitis outbreaks and deaths in the dialysis clinics, and it was known that hepatitis carriers were common among the patients. After Congress passed legislation for federal support of the cost of dialysis, the numbers of U.S. clinics had vastly increased—especially for-profit units, since the Feds guaranteed payment. In an effort to control the spread of disease in dialysis units in Philadelphia, we agreed to monitor their patients for hepatitis carriers. Tom London undertook the responsibility of maintaining this logistically complex project. One day, early in our association with the clinic, Tom was approached by one of the medical staff, who told him that a candidate for dialysis was found to be an HBV carrier. He solicited Tom's advice on what to do. Tom asked what would be the outcome if the patient wasn't accepted for dialysis. The answer was, in effect, that he would die. Tom's immediate response was "Put him on his own dialysis machine and we'll figure out what to do next."[8]

[8] Epidemiological efforts, the establishment of separate dialysis units for HBV carriers, improvements in the sterilization of the dialysis machines, and, later, vaccina-

Even more difficult policy questions arose. For example, while visiting in an eastern European country controlled by a military government, I was asked my opinion on a policy that was being discussed. They were in the process of deciding whether they should block entry to medical school and to military officers' training school for young people who were found to be HBV carriers. People's lives and careers would be determined by the results of the Au test! An even more dramatic difficulty developed. Near the end of the conflict in Vietnam, children, many of whom were orphans, became available for adoption. Mechanisms were set in place to bring them to the United States and other Western countries, where they would undergo adoption processing. HBV carriers are very common in Vietnam; in some of our earliest studies we determined that the carrier rate was 6 percent or greater. Should the children be tested for HBV and those identified as carriers be denied entry to the country or removed from the lists of adoption candidates? Was a child's fate to be determined by the results of this single test? This question was answered differently in different countries. In the United States the U.S. Public Health Service decided not to test for HBV. In other countries the test was required but in many cases was not administered despite the requirement.

These and similar experiences made it clear that we were witnessing the emergence of individuals and classes of people stigmatized by the results of a single laboratory test. The field was in transition; although research was daily hastening the possibilities of prevention, control, and treatment, at the moment there was little that could be done for the carriers or those they associated with. There was a balance between the public good and a possible disadvantage to an individual. In the case of testing blood donors for the presence of carriers, the balance of advantage and disadvantage was clear: the testing spared the transfused patients the obvious disadvantages of hepatitis, while the discomfort to the donors, who were advised not to donate blood again, was not great, at least immediately. However, the testing of the *general* population had little appar-

tion led to the control of these epidemics. Dialysis units are now essentially free of HBV infections.

ent merit, since the control measures were not very effective, and the possible stigmatization of the detected carriers was an obvious disadvantage. On the face of it, the carriers, under normal circumstances, did not appear to be very infectious. There were probably about one million carriers in the United States: if HBV were as infectious as, say, the common cold, there would be far more cases than were known to occur. Several health-care workers who were carriers had been identified, and they did not apparently transmit disease to their patients. There was little benefit to society in general surveys and much disadvantage to the individual.

The consensus of opinion was that research should be hastened, but that no further action on widespread general blood testing should be taken until some good could come of it. As we will see in the next chapter, that happened pretty rapidly after the invention of the vaccine and the improvement in the diagnostic techniques. At that point, the ambiguous state of affairs in respect to carriers was, to a large extent, but not entirely, resolved.

These experiences were an eerie foreshadowing of the problems encountered with the human immunodeficiency virus (HIV) and AIDS, the disease it causes. HBV and HIV are transmitted in a similar manner: by transfusion, sexually, from mother to child, and by contaminated needles. HBV is more infectious and more easily transmitted than HIV, and morbidity and mortality have different patterns. But the problems raised by the social attitudes toward carriers of the viruses are similar, although the consequences have been far more widespread and difficult for HIV. I will have more to say about HIV in later chapters.

The Daedalus Effect

The solution of one problem—the identification of the hepatitis B virus and the (partial) control of posttransfusion hepatitis—raised another problem, the stigmatization of the carriers: the observation was intriguing. Any experienced scientist is aware of the generality of this phenomenon in science. It also was of great practical importance. It is very useful to know that something unexpected will happen—that is, to expect the unexpected—because it increases your sensitivity to eventual trouble and can hasten understanding and solutions of new problems as they arise. At this time, I became fascinated with the metaphor of the mythic Greek artist-scientist Daedalus.[9] I collaborated with a colleague, the brilliant sociologist of clinical research Professor Renée Fox[10] of the University of Pennsylvania, in writing a paper[11] discussing the concept of what we termed the "Daedalus Effect." The myth is long and complex, and I have extracted parts of it as a metaphor for the problem-solving–problem-creating character of science.

In the myth, Daedalus, an Athenian by birth, was an artist, sculptor, and restless inventor and scientist. He settled in Knossos, the glittering capital of Crete, ruled by King Minos and his bride Queen Pasiphae. The king and queen had fallen into serious trouble with the gods. Poseidon had given to Minos a pure white bull of the sea as a sign to the people of Crete that Minos was their rightful king. It was understood that, in time, the bull would be sacrificed to the gods, but Minos admired it so much that he decided to integrate it into his own breeding stock and sacrifice another fine white bull, but not the prize of the gods, in its place. The gods sought revenge. They caused Pasiphae to fall in love with the bull and develop an insatiable desire to have union with it. Daedalus was enlisted in the scheme. His drive to be creative overcame any consideration of the ultimate use and consequences of his invention. He fashioned a hol-

[9] My interest in Daedalus was inspired by my reading of *A Feather for Daedalus*, by Kim Malville (Menlo Park, CA: Cummings, 1975), which carries the Daedalian metaphor much further than I had the courage to carry it.

[10] Renée Fox is a pioneer in the understanding of the sociology of medical research. She has done extensive studies of a variety of research issues, including a long-term analysis of the Belgian research community, including that community's extensive fieldwork in the then Belgian Congo. She and her colleague Ruth Swazey published a pioneering sociological study of the early research programs that resulted in the introduction of kidney transplantation and renal dialysis. It was great working with Renée on the paper. She had a scholar's thoroughness, a respect for the meaning of words that I found overwhelming, and a readily rechargeable sense of humor that made the process of writing the paper a pleasure.

[11] B. S. Blumberg and R. C. Fox, "The Daedalus Effect: Changes in Ethical Questions relating to Hepatitis B Virus," *Annals of Internal Medicine* 102 (1985): 390–94.

low, life-size, internally upholstered model of a cow into which the queen was placed. The contrivance was set in a pasture, where it attracted the great white bull, and the queen's desire was fulfilled.

So the problem was solved, but the solution created another problem—namely, the issue of this union, the half-human, half-beast Minotaur. Because of its savage character, the Minotaur was a catastrophe. Again, Daedalus, the problem solver, was called to assist with the new problem. He invented and had constructed a maze, a labyrinth, in which the man-beast was imprisoned. Another solution—but another problem too. Each year a quota of Athenian young men and women were brought to Crete and sacrificed to the imprisoned monster. Daedalus, himself an Athenian, came to the rescue with still another solution. He told Ariadne, the daughter of Minos and Pasiphae (hence half-sister to the Minotaur), about a secret door into the maze and gave her a simple spool of thread that could be unwound in the passage through the maze, thereby marking the escape route. When the killer-hero Theseus was sent with the putative sacrificial youths to kill the monster, he was befriended by Ariadne; in exchange for his promise to take her away with him when he departed, she gave him the spool and the secrets. Theseus entered the maze, killed the Minotaur, and escaped the labyrinth using the aids provided by his girlfriend; together, they fled. There relationship came to a sticky end when Theseus abandoned Ariadne on Naxos.

Another problem solved, but another problem generated. Minos, angered by the murder of the Minotaur, imprisoned Daedalus and his son Icarus in the maze. What an irony! The maze maker imprisoned in the maze of his own making. But the ever inventive scientist developed a novel vertical solution to his family's problem. He conceptualized a theory of flight, fashioned wings from feathers and wax, and, along with Icarus, flew free. Sadly, Icarus did not heed parental advice and, in his exuberance, flew too close to the sun, lost his wings, and plunged into the sea. Despite his fatherly despair, Daedalus flew on to Cumae, near the metropolis of Naples, and eventually found his way to Sicily—where many sites still commemorate him—to continue his inventions, the solving of some problems and the creation of others.

Daedalus clearly enjoyed his inventions and creations, but he relished the problems as well, perhaps even more than their solutions. His energy and initiative made him appealing to his patrons—at least to a point—and drove Daedalus to seek problems to solve. He might be accused of not thinking through the consequences of his actions in advance, but, in fairness, how could anyone have predicted the actual outcomes at the inception of the solutions? He had learned the ultimate lesson of those who seek to be active in a complex world where experience teaches the frequency of imperfect solutions: that is, the courage to prevail in spite of constant problems.

# The Hepatitis B Vaccine

THE MOST SIGNIFICANT outcome of our research has, probably, been the invention and the introduction of the hepatitis B vaccine, one of the most widely used vaccines in the world and the first "cancer vaccine."[1] By "cancer vaccine," I mean an agent that can *prevent* cancer—in this case, one of the most common cancers in the world, primary cancer of the liver. In this chapter, I will relate the story of our invention of the vaccine and the events that led to its manufacture, testing, and acceptance for general use. The apparent success of the HBV vaccine in the prevention of primary cancer of the liver (of which I will write more later) has encouraged the search for other vaccines for cancer prevention, a very hopeful step in the control of this widespread and feared group of diseases.

In early 1969, at one of the staff council meetings of the Institute for Cancer Research, Tim Talbot, then director, told us a piece of unwelcome news. He had been informed by the National Cancer Institute that in the future, support would be diminished and applicant institutions would be expected to seek additional sources of money elsewhere. The implication was that we should try to patent and commercialize the products of our research. (I remind the

---

[1] There is a great deal of focus currently on the development of "cancer vaccines," which often means vaccines that can be used to *treat* an already existing cancer. With the possible exception of a vaccine to treat malignant melanoma (whose effectiveness is not entirely clear) and several experimental vaccines based on new concepts from molecular biology, there are no therapeutic vaccines in common use for cancers.

reader that this was years before the advent of molecular biology and the entrepreneurial biotechnology industry that it engendered, which has turned many scientists into businesspersons.) As it turned out, I do not think that this threat was actualized, and the generous funding from the federal government continued for several more years. At the time, though, we could only assume that our funding was in jeopardy. The notion that a principal source of research support might be constrained, like the prospect of hanging, can sharply focus the mind. Action was needed.

I spoke to Irv Millman and told him that we had to file a patent for a hepatitis B vaccine. We had been thinking about this matter ever since our first population studies; even though the virus had been discovered barely two years earlier, and we had only just started the testing of donor blood in the hospitals, we started on the invention of the vaccine. I was unburdened by any preconceived ideas as to how a vaccine should be made, although I had a general knowledge from medical school of the theory of their production and use. Irv, on the other hand, had considerable experience. He had worked at the vaccine facility of the Merck Institute for Therapeutic Research in West Point, a suburb of Philadelphia. He had had no experience of hepatitis there but did invent and patent a purified pertussis vaccine superior to any others then available. Unfortunately, Merck decided not to produce it, and that, in part, was the reason that Irv came to work with us. He thought, when we first recruited him, that he would be working on serum protein polymorphisms, but by the time he arrived we were well into the hepatitis caper, and Irv was drawn back into infectious disease research.

Regardless of my inexperience with the invention of vaccines, I had a keen perception of the value of public health and preventive medicine. In Suriname, in Africa, in the central Pacific, and indeed in Alaska—the venues of much of my early research—I had witnessed the paramount importance of public health measures, including vaccination. Much of the disease in developing parts of the world could be prevented if the water and food supply were safeguarded from contamination by human waste, if insect vectors for viruses, parasites, and other infectious agents were controlled, and and if childhood vaccination were routinely implemented.

What was the evidence that we could make a vaccine? It was thin, but compelling. One of the big problems in making a vaccine is identifying the protective antibody—that is, a gamma globulin protein present in the blood of an immunized person, or a specific reaction of the immune cells that would protect against infection with a specific infectious agent.[2] Much of the concern about developing a vaccine for HIV, the causative agent for AIDS, is centered on this issue. The molecular biology of HIV is well understood, probably better than any other virus that has ever been identified, but the protective antigens and mechanisms are not known. This makes it very difficult for scientists to decide which antigen to use for the vaccine. However, from the very beginning of the research on HBV, there were very good indications about what must be the protective antibody. The data were pretty simple: in our early tests on thousands of individual sera, we had rarely seen a person who had HBsAg in the blood—that is, was a carrier of HBV—and, at the same time, had the antibody against the surface antigen (anti-HBs). This is consistent with the hypothesis that anti-HBs is protective against infection. The problem was further simplified by the stark reality that anti-HBs was the only known antibody. Providentially, the first antibody we knew was the one that protects.

There were ancillary data. During the course of our earlier studies at Philadelphia General Hospital and elsewhere, we noted that transfused patients who had the antibody before transfusion, or developed it after transfusion, were less likely to experience hepatitis events than patients who did not. This was also the conclusion of Okochi's published paper to which I have already referred. The amounts of data were not large, but they were statistically significant. In a previous chapter, I described the experiments with the vervet monkeys demonstrating that Au could be transmitted to an

---

[2] Antibodies are glycoproteins—that is, proteins with sugars attached to them—that are produced by the immune systems of vertebrates. They are essential in the defense of the host against invasion by microorganisms. The glycoproteins are highly variable in composition, and they can recognize specific molecular groupings on the microorganisms, or on other proteins or biochemicals to which the immune system may be exposed. Any molecule bound specifically to an antibody is termed an antigen; antigens can come from many sources, including microorganisms.

experimental animal. This experiment also provided invaluable information toward the invention of the vaccine. The purified particles that contained only the surface antigen (HBsAg), which were very common in the blood, could be separated from the infectious particles—which were rare—by centrifugation. The purified particles, without the infectious material, did not transmit HBV to the vervets, whereas the less purified material, which contained the infectious material, did do so.

In the patent application we described a method for separating the HBsAg particles using centrifugation in various media, such as sugar solution or cesium chloride, and applying enzymes to remove any serum protein remaining and also to impair or destroy any viable virus that might remain, followed by column separation and treatment by several methods to kill residual virus of any kind. Substances to increase the antigenicity of the HBsAg—that is, to increase the ability of the vaccine to elicit a protective response from the vaccinated person—and preservatives to increase shelf life could be added—and *voilà*, the vaccine. Under the electron microscope we could see the small particles (similar to those visualized earlier by Manfred Bayer, Barbara Werner, and me) in large numbers and densely packed. We filed with the U.S. Patent Office on 8 October 1969, and the patent was issued, without much hassle, on 18 January 1972.

Ours was a unique method for making a vaccine. None had been prepared in this manner before, and none have been since. There are several processes for making vaccines. The first vaccine, against smallpox, consisted of the human virus contained in the fluid extruded from the pustules of a person who had been mildly infected. The notion was that a person would be more likely to survive a controlled infection than a natural one, and that this induced infection would provide protection against subsequent natural infections that might be more serious. That may have been true, but the mortality rate from vaccination with the human virus was unacceptably high, of the order of 10 percent. Edward Jenner's (1749–1823) original contribution came when he noted that milkmaids had better complexions than other women: they did not bear the facial scarring that follows recovery from human smallpox. Milkmaids were prone to infection with cowpox virus, an infectious agent in cattle similar to human smallpox. Why didn't the milkmaids succumb to smallpox? Cowpox does not cause serious or fatal illness in humans, and the scarring is much less severe than with human smallpox. Jenner theorized that infection with cowpox somehow prevented infection with the human virus. He administered the cowpox virus[3] as a preventive vaccine, and it achieved great success, although its use was by no means unmarred by controversy. For example, there were objections on what were considered by some to be religious grounds. It was argued that using the preventive measures would thwart God's will. The word "vaccine," derived from the Latin root *vacca* (as in the French *vache*), is a reminder of the bovine origins of the first vaccine.

Scientists have created other vaccines through a process of "attenuating" natural infectious agents—that is, decreasing their ability to cause disease—by transmitting them serially through experimental animals or through tissue cultures. The Sabin polio vaccine is of this nature. Such vaccines can be administered easily, by mouth (some readers will remember taking a sugar cube with a few drops of vaccine on it). Further, because they are infectious, they can spread to members of the community who have not been vaccinated—each individual vaccination thus has an amplified effect. The disadvantage is that some people become ill from the attenuated vaccine, and deaths occasionally occur. These are very infrequent; when polio was a terrible scourge, the risk from the use of the vaccine to a few members of the population warranted its use in the population as a whole. But when polio became rare, as it is now, there were in some communities more cases of illness due to the vaccine than to natural infection.

Killed vaccines are another option. Scientists create these by taking the offending virus or other microorganism, killing it by heating or by some chemical process, and then using the resulting denatured, but antigenic, protein as the vaccine. (The Salk polio vaccine

---

[3] The identity of the virus that was administered in the vaccine gradually drifted away from the original cowpox used by Jenner, probably because of the introduction of other viruses as well as natural evolution of the original strain.

was made this way.) Sometimes the whole organism is used and sometimes only a portion of it. With the advent of molecular biology it has become possible to be precisely selective, and to clone a gene from the virus for a particular antigen and produce only that as a vaccine. Even fancier vaccines are now being designed—for example, DNA vaccines in which the DNA that produces the desired protein is injected into the host and the vaccine antigen is produced by the host.

Our vaccine wasn't made by any of these processes. Rather, we took antigen from individuals who had a great deal of it and used it to inoculate others who didn't have any: a "people's vaccine," as we sometimes jokingly called it. Our ability to do this was based on the fact that the virus produced very large quantities of the small, noninfectious particles containing only the surface antigen. This was probably an immunologic strategy of the virus, producing excess amounts of the antigen in the blood to divert the antibodies produced by the host's immune system to the small particles and thereby to spare the whole virus, which could get on with its mischief of replication and damage to the liver cells. In the war parlance of the infectious disease field, this is sometimes referred to as a "smoke screen."

The vaccine was invented. What were we to do next? To transform the vaccine from a theory to an actuality, we had to interest a pharmaceutical manufacturer in the project. FCCC was not set up to produce and test a vaccine. The equipment needed to maintain production standards required for a vaccine to be used in humans was not available in a research laboratory, nor did we wish to redirect the basic science activities of the institution. In 1969, when we first invented the vaccine, there was little faith in the hepatitis community or among the pharmaceutical companies that we had identified the virus—much less produced, by a totally unconventional method, a vaccine that would be practical and economically profitable. There was another issue that probably diminished interest in the vaccine. Hepatitis was not considered to be a serious disease in the developed world. In most people's experience, it was a very unpleasant acute disease that lasted for a few days or weeks, and from which recovery was nearly always complete. Also, it was regarded as primarily a disease of other places, one that you might encounter on a holiday visit to the tropics, or that was contracted overseas by people in the military. The long-term consequences of infection, chronic liver disease and cancer of the liver, were not known until the Au test and its improvements were available to show the connection.

There were several developments that moved matters forward. In April 1970 Dr. Saul Krugman, professor of pediatrics at New York University, and his colleagues reported a series of experiments that drew attention to the possibilities of the vaccine. They boiled serum containing Australia antigen for one minute and used it as a vaccine to inoculate Down's syndrome children, who were then given un-boiled serum containing Australia antigen. The boiled serum appeared to confer some, but not complete, protection against subsequent exposure. Although these experiments were criticized on ethical grounds, and were faulted to some extent scientifically as well (in the initial experiments there were no controls), they did have the effect of impressing scientists and vaccine manufacturers as to the possibility of a vaccine.

There was also additional evidence that anti-HBs was effective. Beginning in November 1970 Tom London had been monitoring and attempting, with a great deal of success, to prevent the development of hepatitis in renal dialysis units in Philadelphia. Ed Lust-bader executed a fascinating analysis of the mass of data Tom had collected over several years. It was originally presented at a meeting in Paris and published in French;[4] it was later published in more complete form in English.[5] He compared the probability of *not* developing hepatitis in initially uninfected renal dialysis patients who entered with anti-HBs in their blood to that of patients who did lacked the substance. The differences were impressive (fig. 5): after nine months of treatment on the dialysis unit (usually about three visits a week), only 50 percent of the patients who did not have anti-

[4] B. S. Blumberg, W. T. London, E. D. Lustbader, J. S. Drew, and B. G. Werner, "Protection vis-à-vis de l'hepatite B par l'anti-HBs chez des malades hemodialyses. *Hepatite à Virus B t Hemodialyse* (Paris: Flammarion Médecine-Sciences, 1975), 175–83.

[5] E. D. Lustbader, W. T. London, and B. S. Blumberg, "Study Design for a Hepatitis B Vaccine Trial," *Proceedings of the National Academy of Sciences* 73 (1976): 955–59.

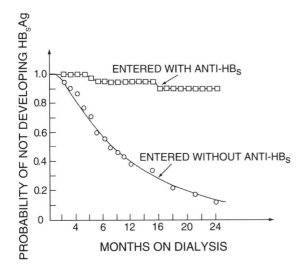

Fig. 5. The probability of not developing HBsAg over the course of twenty-four months in renal dialysis patients admitted with and without anti-HBs. The anti-HBs is highly effective in preventing infection. (Lustbader, London, and Blumberg, *Proceedings of the National Academy of Sciences* 73 [1976]: 955–59.)

HBs on entry remained uninfected, while of those who entered with anti-HBs, more than 90 percent remained uninfected. This was a dramatic illustration of the protective property of the antibody that could be produced by the vaccine. Additionally, by the mid-1970s a series of experimental studies done on primates in several laboratories appeared to show that the vaccine was protective, confirming the preliminary findings on animal inoculation that had been presented in the vaccine patent application.

By 1971 we were in discussion with the scientists at Merck & Co., whose facility for vaccine research was located in West Point, Pennsylvania, not far from Philadelphia, and they expressed an interest in licensing the vaccine. Nothing much happened immediately. The scientific community was still testing the hypothesis that our research was really valid, and that we had identified the virus that causes hepatitis B. We had spoken and written about our concept for the vaccine and discussed it with colleagues in the hepatitis field, but it still required more research and confirmation by others. Research on hepatitis B has never been very well funded, and there were not many investigators in the field to do the necessary studies. It took time for the subsequent steps to unfold.

The federal government had decided, strangely, to grant us ownership of the foreign, but not the domestic, rights to the patent. This compelled Irv Millman and me to seriously dedicate ourselves to identifying a company we could license. In 1975 we traveled to Europe for discussions with British and French pharmaceutical companies. In Paris, we met with the elder Dr. Merrioux, whose company was one of the major producers of vaccines in France, and he and his son expressed interest in acquiring the rights to the vaccine. This could have been a satisfactory arrangement, but we decided that, if possible, a domestic manufacturer would be better—not only because of proximity but because we had been supported by U.S. tax funds (and, to a limited extent, funds from the Commonwealth of Pennsylvania), and, if the vaccine became a commercially valuable product, the economic advantage should if possible be national and local. To that end, I drove up to Rahway, New Jersey, the headquarters of the Merck corporation, with G. Willing Pepper (known as "Wing") to speak with the chief operating officer of the company. Wing was the chairman of the Board of Trustees of Fox Chase Cancer Center, a war hero (a four-striper in the Navy, he had been aboard the carrier USS *Wasp* when it was sunk during the Battle of Guadalcanal), and himself the retired CEO of a large Philadelphia company. The conversation between Wing and the Merck CEO seemed to be an amiable discussion about mutual friends, with occasional laughing references to the patent and its value. There didn't seem to be any closure by the time we left the room. Perhaps I was distracted by the opulence of the office and reception area; I remember thinking at the time that we could easily fit four good-size laboratory spaces into the room occupied by a single executive. The proceedings seemed to be inconclusive and somewhat depressing. When we emerged from the building, I said to Wing. "Well, I guess that was 'No.'" "To the contrary," Wing answered, "it was 'Yes.'" So much for my appreciation of corporate dealings.

In 1975 FCCC licensed Merck to develop the vaccine. Dr. Maurice Hilleman, who had considerable experience in the development and manufacture of vaccines and in hepatitis research, was the executive in charge of the program. Merck was very effective, and soon they had sufficient knowledge of the vaccine, and a sufficient quantity of it, to undertake field trials.

Dr. Wolf Szmuness and his colleagues in New York City conducted the first formal trial published.[6] It was a very well designed and well executed study, and we and all the beneficiaries of the vaccine owe a great deal to Wolf for producing a study so convincing that it probably speeded up the acceptance of the vaccine by more than a year. Wolf was an interesting man who had surmounted many difficulties in his career and life. He and his family were caught up in the turmoil of the German invasion of Poland at the start of World War II, and they fled to the east. He was educated in the Soviet Union and returned to Poland after the war. After his medical training, he became a public health physician and had experience administering and testing vaccines in his homeland. In the 1960s, there was a series of pogroms directed against the remnant of the Jewish population in Poland that had survived the war, and Wolf and his family fled again, this time to the United States. He visited our laboratory, and we discussed the possibility of an appointment for him. However—probably wisely, as it turned out—he decided to work at the New York Blood Center, from where he organized the field trial for our HBV vaccine.

First, Wolf wanted to identify a population at high risk for hepatitis. The early clinical and epidemiological studies had given us some idea of the methods of transmission. These included mother-to-child, sexual, transfusion, and use of contaminated injection needles. Individuals with impaired immune responses were particularly susceptible. The subsequent work on HIV, which is transmitted by the same methods as HBV (but is less infectious), has made the public very aware of the mechanisms by which blood-borne viruses are spread. Populations that had a high probability of becoming infected with HBV were pretty well known and have already been discussed. These included the Down's syndrome patients, Hansen's

---

[6] W. Szmuness, C. E. Stevens, E. J. Harley, et al., "Hepatitis B Vaccine: Demonstration of Efficacy in a Controlled Clinical Trial in a High-Risk Population in the United States," *New England Journal of Medicine* 303 (1980): 833–41.

disease patients, renal dialysis patients, and others. Some of the first carriers we encountered were members of the homosexual community in Philadelphia, and, at a clinical level, it was known that hepatitis was common in this population. Wolf and his colleagues did a systematic study in the New York City gay male community and found that the rate of infection was very high. In a sample of about ten thousand people, he found the prevalence of serological markers of HBV infection to be 68 percent, very much higher than in other segments of the population. He also estimated the annual incidence rate—that is, the percentage of people who became infected within a year—and found that it was nearly 20 percent. Wolf told me that in subsequent studies it was even higher; as many as a third of those previously uninfected would become so within a year. It also became apparent that the members of this community were well educated, intelligent, and willing to volunteer for a research project that could benefit themselves and others. He decided to enlist their cooperation to test the vaccine.[7]

To obtain the necessary statistical power, he required about 400 individuals who would receive the vaccine and an additional 400 who would receive a placebo. In the event, between November 1978 and October 1979, 1,083 individuals (549 vaccine, 534 placebo) were enrolled in the trial. On the basis of random selection individuals were designated to receive either the vaccine or the placebo, and each was assigned an identifying code. The recipients did not know whether they received vaccine or placebo, and the physicians who were to do the evaluation also did not know. The code was retained, to be connected with a name only after the studies were complete. The vaccine was administered in three doses, the first two one month apart and the third six months after the first. Ninety-three percent of the subjects received all three inoculations, an indication of the excellent compliance and the loyalty of the subjects. They were evaluated for the occurrence of a hepatitis event for at least six months; most were followed for a year. What happened?

---

[7] The major use of HBV vaccine has been and will be in Asia, Africa, and the Pacific. However, the initial tests establishing safety and efficacy were done in the United States. In this case, Americans were the initial site of testing for the rest of the world's population.

When the code was broken, the results were impressive. First, there was no difference in deleterious side effects between those who had been given the placebo and those who had received the vaccine. As far as I can tell, in the many years since this first trial and after a billion doses of vaccine have been administered, although concerns have been raised,[8] there is still no convincing evidence of detrimental side effects due to the vaccine. Second, the response to the vaccine was excellent. Ninety-six percent of those vaccinated developed antibody after completing the three-dose regimen. Third, there was a striking difference between the vaccinated and the controls with respect to the development of hepatitis B. A total of fifty-two individuals developed hepatitis B as scored by chemical abnormalities and the appearance of HBsAg in the blood. Only seven of these were in the vaccinated group, and of these only one had completed the full course of vaccination. It is likely that some of these vaccinated people had actually been infected shortly before the vaccinations began. There was an additional finding of great clinical importance. The vaccinated people who did not develop anti-HBs did not become carriers of HBV more frequently than those who received placebo. Had this not been the case, then our findings would have raised the possibility that persons who were destined to become carriers, possibly because of an inherited propensity to do so, would not respond to vaccination. If this were true, then a

---

[8] On 27 April 1998 an ABC news story raised concerns about the safety of the HBV vaccine. On 30 April the Centers for Disease Control in Atlanta posted a note on their website conveying reassurances of safety. These were further discussed in the 31 July 1998 issue of *Science* (E. Marshall, "A Shadow Falls on Hepatitis B Vaccination Effort," *Science* 281 [1998]: 630–31). It stated, in part, "A growing number of people who have received the vaccine shots—although just a tiny fraction of the two hundred million immunized—claim to have experienced serious adverse effects." Most of what were believed to be side effects were related to autoimmune and arthritic disorders, neurological symptoms, and multiple sclerosis (MS). The author then noted that there was little evidence to support this contention, and the available studies did not show that toxicity was an issue. In May 1999 Dr. David Margolis of the CDC reported to a committee of the U.S. House of Representatives on the question of HBV vaccine side effects. He cited several studies that demonstrated safety, and, specifically, noted that the research ruled against the possibility that HBV vaccination was related to multiple sclerosis and sudden infant death syndrome. By mid-2000 the concern appeared to have abated.

major value of the vaccine would have been lost. But the results reported by Wolf and the others taught that this was not the case, and that it would be possible to vaccinate even those who were at greater risk of becoming carriers. This conclusion was supported in a study in South Africa that showed, for the first time, that vaccinated infants who were born of carrier mothers, and were known to be at great risk of becoming carriers, did develop anti-HBs and were protected against infection and the carrier state.

There were subsequent field trials that also supported the efficacy of the vaccine. Within two years of the publication of Wolf's paper, in the early 1980s, the FDA approved the blood-derived vaccine, and within a few years, millions of children and adults were being vaccinated yearly. (In 2000 it was estimated that a billion doses of the vaccine had been administered.) It is now one of the most commonly used vaccines in the world.

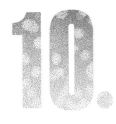 **Hepatitis B Virus and Cancer of the Liver**

THE MOST IMPORTANT practical outcome of research on hepatitis B has been the campaign to prevent primary cancer of the liver, one of the most common and deadly cancers in the world. The early reports on the outcome of this campaign are very promising. If they are supported in the future, the world is well on its way to a new and effective method for the prevention of cancer. Primary cancer of the liver is not the only cancer linked to a virus, and the research on HBV and liver cancer may provide a guide to the prevention of other cancers in the future.

What were the events that have led to this happy progress? In this chapter, I will describe our role in the program.

Uganda

July 1971. The skyline of Budapest was shrinking into the distance behind us as the hydrofoil proceeded at a comfortable pace westward along the Danube towards Vienna. It occurred to me that this was a curious route to East Africa. I had spent several days at a meeting on tropical medicine in Hungary (it seemed an unusual place for this subject); I was on my way to Kampala in Uganda to attend meetings on cancer in Africa and to start our studies on the transmission of HBV by insects. Budapest still retained the grandeur of its days as the second capital of the Austro-Hungarian Empire, but the predominant effect was the colorless and rundown character of a behind-the-Iron-Curtain communist city. However, during the sunny days of summer, the streets had been filled with informally dressed people, the young men and women in shorts and jeans demonstrating their cultural and emotional affinities with the West in the unspoken language of appearance.

The hydrofoil skirted the Czechoslovakian city of Bratislava; there had been rumors in Budapest of demonstrations against the Soviet presence in the country, but all seemed peaceful as we sailed by. Vienna lived up to its reputation as a beautifully preserved and enhanced city. The famous opera house, the pride of the city, which had been rebuilt after its destruction during the Second World War, was magnificent. But I did not sense the intellectual excitement the city had known when it was a hotbed of activity in the interwar period. I visited the Allegemaine Krankenhaus, the famous university teaching hospital, which in past decades housed many of the famous physicians and scientists of the period when German-speaking medical schools were the model for academic medicine.

I boarded the Sabena aircraft at Vienna International and sped through the night into Africa. We landed in Entebbe the next morning, entering Uganda at a fateful time in the history of that beautiful country; it was just after the accession of Idi Amin to the leadership after Milton Obote had been ousted during a visit abroad. This was followed by a protracted period of unrest and bloody civil war, a terrible deterrent to the health and development of the country. The unrest was not yet manifest, or at least not obvious, when we arrived for the meeting. It was difficult to know what was happening because journalists were not permitted to print the news freely. Friends at the hospital told us that many wounded soldiers had been admitted for treatment. The rumor was that there were political and intertribal battles in the barracks, with many fatalities and injuries. Later, when I was in the backcountry collecting mosquitoes, I had an uncomfortable run-in with the authorities. I was taken into the police post in a small town and questioned by plainclothes officers who appeared suspicious and even hostile. I was released when I assured them I had not taken any pictures of the police station, and destroyed the exposed film I had in my camera. It was only after I returned to the United States that I learned that two foreign

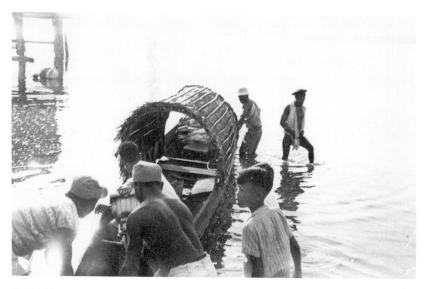

1. The Marowyne River, Suriname, October 1950. The *corrial*, or log dugout canoe, that we used to travel upriver (south) from Albina, near the mouth of the river, to Langatabatje, the main settlement of the Paramacanner nation. There was a crew of four paddlers, boat handlers, and assistants and a medical team of three. We used an outboard motor in slack water but had to paddle or haul the boat through the shoals and rapids.

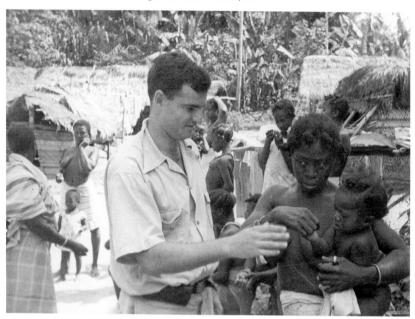

2. Suriname. Clinical examinations in a riverside village near Moengo. In addition to collecting specimens for the malaria, filaria, and other surveys, we conducted daily clinics, medical and dental, under the supervision of Dr. Ian Guicherit, the physician for the Moengo region. There were no roads and few paths connecting these communities, and all travel was by river.

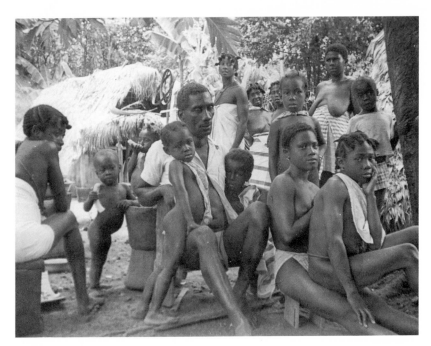

3. Suriname. A village group awaiting a visit with the mobile clinic staff. The houses were made of local wood, usually elaborately carved in a distinctive style. The roofs were of thatch, and the houses were often raised above the ground to safeguard them from the flooding that occurred in the rainy season.

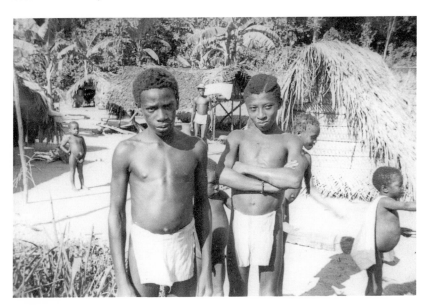

4. Suriname. Village youths in the reception party at Langatabatje. The usual dress was a covering of the lower part of the body and sometimes a toga-like cape partially covering the upper torso.

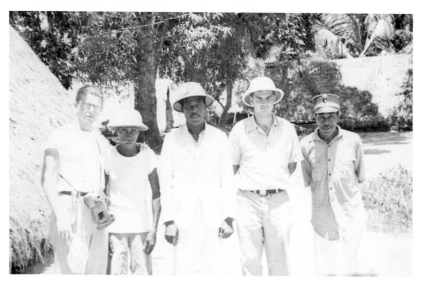

5. Suriname. John McGiff (far left), a medical school classmate of mine at the College of Physicians and Surgeons, Columbia University, and me (second from right) with the *Granman* of the Paramacanners in the Marowyne River island community of Langatabatje. We conducted several days of *palavar*—that is, extended discussions—with the *Granman* and his staff concerning our medical surveys and treatment program. We were camped on the riverside near his town and paddled over daily for our meetings.

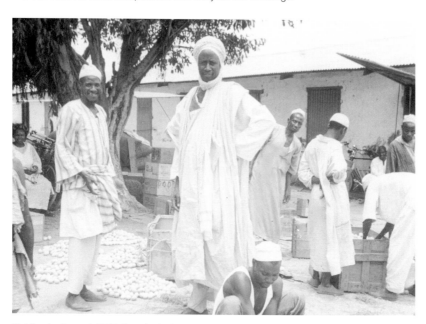

6. Nigeria, August 1957. A trader in the marketplace. The markets were the centers of activity in many of the communities, and our visits would usually start there. The medical studies were done in a clinic or other public building near the market.

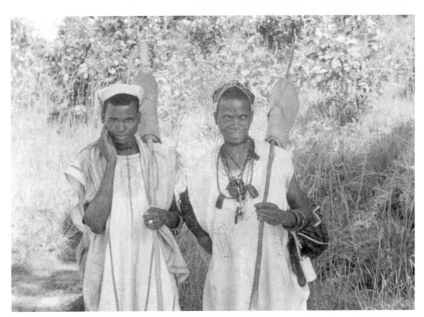

7. Nigeria, August 1957. Two Fulani men on their way to town. The Fulani ordinarily lived in semipermanent camps in rural areas adjacent to a larger community. It was often difficult to locate their encampments; we would go the nearest village, ask in the marketplace where they might be, and then head into the bush looking for them. In this case we encountered these young men who guided us to their homes.

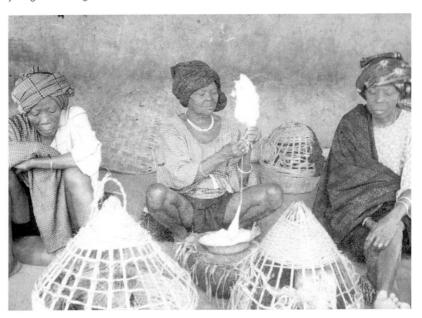

8. Nigeria, 1957. Market women spinning cotton with a distaff. Many of the merchants were women and were important sources of information on the medical and other resources in the community.

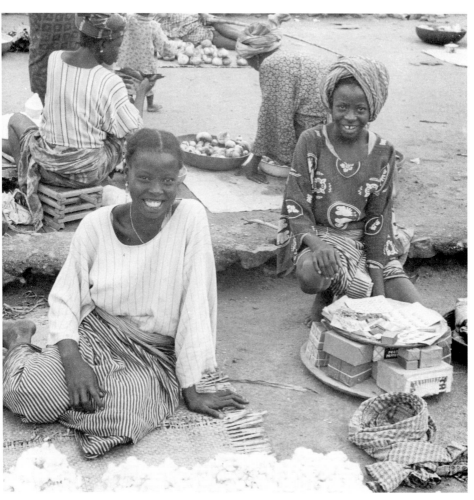

9. Nigeria, 1957. Another view of a marketplace.

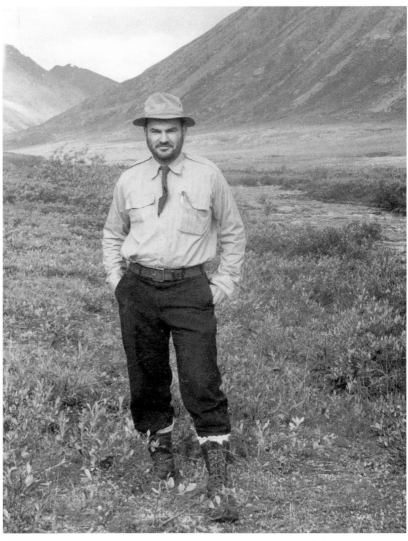

10. Alaska, August 1958. Anaktuvuk Pass in the Brooks Range, northern Alaska, the home of an isolated group of Inuits. I was dressed for a meeting with the village leaders to explain the research program and the purpose of our visit.

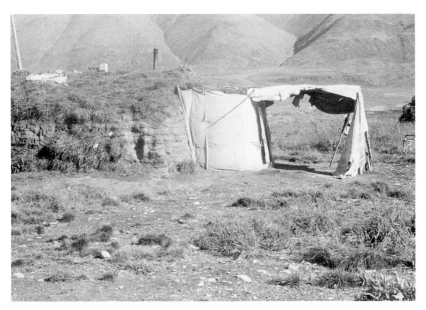

11. Alaska, August 1958, Anaktuvuk Pass. Turf and canvas igloo used during the summer months. Traditional living styles were still in evidence in this remote community, but they were rapidly changing. While we were in the pass, wooden frame houses were being built to replace these traditional homes.

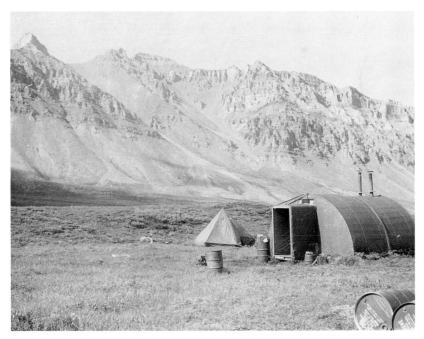

12. Alaska, August 1958. Quonset hut on the shores of the pond at Anaktuvuk Pass where the medical field party camped. The plane landed on the small pond beyond the hut.

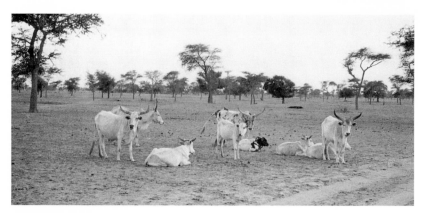

13. Senegal, 1976. Many of the medical studies in Senegal were done in the village complex of Tip, located two hundred kilometers east of Dakar. The setting was pastoral but arid, except for the rainy season. Cattle grazed on sparse cropland and pasture.

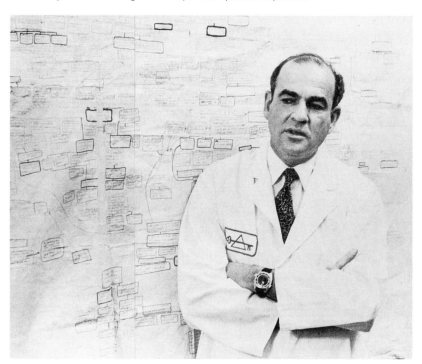

14. In June 1973, while I was on sabbatical at Oxford University, Professor Hans Krebs, the noted biochemist and Nobel laureate, encouraged me to write an account of my research. I started to do so at Oxford and continued the process over the next few years at the Center for Advanced Study in the Behavioral Sciences at Stanford University and at Fox Chase Cancer Center, Philadelphia. I charted the research process in terms of the observations that were first made, the hypotheses that derived from them, the study design required to test the hypotheses, the results of the hypothesis testing, and the new hypotheses that were derived from these. In a sense all the experiments and observations were connected to each other, and the enormous diagram that derived from this is shown, in part, in the background. This analysis was used as the background for the present book. The photograph was taken at Fox Chase Cancer Center, Philadelphia.

journalists (including one from Philadelphia) had been killed near where I had been detained and at about the same time.

Despite these contretemps, the visit to Uganda was to have a profound effect on the direction of my work and that of my colleagues for the next decade. It focused our thinking and research on what is probably the most important outcome of all our work on HBV: the possibility of preventing one of the most common cancers of the world, primary cancer of the liver, by the use of the HBV vaccine—the first effective "cancer vaccine."

Primary hepatocellular carcinoma is a cancer that originates in the liver. This distinguishes it from cancers that start in other organs (for example, lung, colon, prostate) and then metastasize—that is, spread—to the liver. The term "hepatocellular carcinoma" (abbreviated HCC) also emphasizes that it originates in the liver cells that perform the major functions of the organ, rather than other cells, such as the bile duct cells, that are also present in the liver. The cancer process may start in the liver cells of a susceptible person at a very young age; the affected cells initially divide and reproduce themselves very slowly. (We now know what we only inferred at the time of my visit to Uganda: that the liver cells of those fated to develop HCC were very likely to be infected with HBV. After the discovery of the hepatitis C virus [HCV] it was recognized that this virus, either by itself or in conjunction with HBV, could also be causative.) This slow growth proceeds over many decades, unknown to its host and without any symptoms. When symptoms finally do appear, often several decades after HBV infection, the patient may die within a few months or years. HCC usually occurs in people who already have liver disease, typically due to HBV or HCV. Abdominal pain, weight loss, a mass in the right upper part of the abdomen, and an otherwise unexplained deterioration in the general condition of the patient are indicators that cancer is present. Occasionally, the first indication may be a sudden event such as the rupture of the tumor, or bleeding from a vascular mass. The five-year survival rate[1] after clinical diagnosis is about 5 percent, one of the lowest for any cancer. Treatment of advanced HCC is unsatisfac-

---

[1] Five-year survival means the percentage of people surviving five years after the diagnosis has been made or the treatment completed.

tory, and survival after treatment does not greatly exceed the survival rate for untreated cases. I remember, vividly, an episode when Tom London and I were visiting a provincial hospital in northern Senegal near the Mauretanian border and attended a party hosted by the local physicians. A surgeon, nearly in tears, told us that he had for many years been surgically removing livers filled with advanced cancer, and how little effect this had had on the survival of his patients. He encouraged us to keep up with our research and hoped that it would relieve the suffering that he had unsuccessfully fought for so long.

Worldwide, HCC it is the third most common cause of death from cancer in men and the seventh most common cause in women.[2] In Asia and sub-Saharan Africa, it is a disease of major public health importance. It has been difficult to estimate the yearly number of deaths from HCC partly because cancer registries are not common or comprehensive in many areas where it is most prevalent. Using the available data from cancer registries and hospitals, and extrapolating from detailed statistics from high-incidence areas in China, reported by Tom London in 1997, we can deduce that there may be as many as a million deaths a year from this dreaded disease. It is estimated that about 85 percent of cases of HCC are due to HBV. If one adds to this figure the number of deaths from other outcomes of HBV infection (liver failure due to chronic HBV infection, acute fulminant hepatitis, etc.), the annual deaths attributable to HBV are probably on the order of 1.5 million.[3] It is heartrending to see people in the later stages of HCC and to know that there is little that can be done to treat them. Imagine our growing excitement over the next few years when we realized that we might be able to prevent an enormous amount of misery through the use of the vaccine against HBV.

I came to Uganda to attend an international meeting on cancer in Africa organized by the Uganda Cancer Center, located near the medical school and hospital of Makarere University, the oldest and

---

[2] This disparity in disease rate may seem strange, but in nearly every aspect of the natural and pathological history of HCC there are gender differences. It is a very curious story that will unwind as the book continues.

[3] This is about the yearly number of deaths attributed to the human immunodeficiency virus (HIV), the causative organism of AIDS.

probably the most distinguished medical school in East Africa. The Uganda Cancer Center was funded in large part by the National Cancer Institute of the United States. It might be asked why the United States should fund research in a country distant from our shores and, at least on the face of it, not of immediate health concern to Americans. But these were the days of ample support for medical research. The U.S. research community recognized that the search for knowledge of the mechanisms of cancer should be pursued wherever it could best be done; disease, they recognized, transcends borders. The solution of a medical problem in Africa would be of immediate pertinence to Africans but would also, in time, be of benefit to the general medical community. This is obviously true in the case of infectious diseases that can spread from country to country with the speed of a jet airplane. But it is also relevant to the transfer of ideas about disease from one nation to another.

One day of the conference was devoted to cancer of the liver. It included a series of papers on the association of HBV with HCC. We knew about this work; Bruce Smith[4] and I had already published a paper on the subject. In 1969, only two years after our first publication on HBV, we studied the interconnection of HBV, cancer of the liver, and chronic liver disease.[5] We formulated the hypothesis that HBV (identified by the presence of Australia antigen) caused HCC.[6] The hypothesis was not supported by the data; we did not find a higher incidence of Au in the retrospective study described in the report. ("Retrospective" means that we tested patients who had already developed HCC and compared them to controls who had not.) We now know that the technique we were using for identifying

[4] Bruce was an M.D. who had graduated from medical school in North Carolina. He did part of his postdoctoral clinical training in Philadelphia and then elected to spend several years in research training in my laboratory. Bruce was a dedicated scientist, his intensity nicely balanced by a good sense of humor.

[5] J. B. Smith and B. S. Blumberg, "Viral Hepatitis, Post-necrotic Cirrhosis and Hepatocellular Carcinoma," *Lancet* 2 (1969): 953.

[6] The association of chronic liver disease with cancer of the liver had been recognized since the 1950s but could not readily be tested because HBV had not been identified. According to a WHO review of the subject (*IARC Monographs on the Evaluation of Carcinogenic Risks to Humans*, vol. 59, *Hepatitis Viruses* (Lyons: IARC, 1994), the Smith and Blumberg paper was, apparently, the first in which this hypothesis was articulated.

the virus, immunodiffusion, was too insensitive. When patients who have been carriers of HBV develop cancer of the liver, there is a gradual decrease in the amount of virus in the peripheral blood as the disease advances. Most of the cases included in our study were advanced, and the virus levels had dropped below the detection horizon of our method. In our paper we suggested that the virus might be present in detectable amounts early in the disease but not later. We recommended that additional tests of association should be done. Probably independent of anything we had said, studies were completed during the next few years, and several were presented at the meeting.

Recently, I looked through the notes I took in Kampala and found a table that summarized the surveys from the United States, Uganda, Kenya, Senegal, Hong Kong, Singapore, Japan, Greece, and England. Most of these studies were based on small numbers, and the conclusions were not completely consistent, but in a majority there was a higher prevalence of the virus in the cancer cases than in the controls. Confirming a hypothesis under very different circumstances (e.g., different geography, culture, climate, etc.) is far more impressive than exactly repeating a study. In the multiple-site strategy one can argue that, despite very different conditions, the relation between the variables of concern is so strong that it persists in the presence of other interacting variables. In any case, it convinced many others and us that the study of cancer of the liver and HBV was the way to go. I returned to Philadelphia energized by the meeting and the excitement of Africa itself, and determined to press on with the cancer studies and to encourage others to do so. I also had a suitcase full of frozen mosquitoes collected in the bush, which we tested for the presence of HBV. I will discuss this aspect of the work in the next chapter.

France, Senegal, and Mali

Early in 1973, while I was on sabbatical leave at the Laboratory of Genetics in the Department of Biochemistry at Oxford, Bernard Larouze came from Paris to visit me in my office in an alcove

in the balcony overlooking the tea room. Bernard had been dis-
patched by Professor M. Payet, formerly the dean of the medical
school at the University of Dakar in Senegal, West Africa, and now
at L'Hôpital Claude Bernard in Paris, to suggest that we collaborate
on a study of HBV and HCC. In 1956 Professor Payet and colleagues
had reported a study of more than two hundred cases of HCC seen
in Dakar in what was still colonial Senegal.[7] They found a strong
correlation with liver disease that, on pathological grounds, they believed was caused by infectious hepatitis. The following year
P. Steiner and J. N. Davies published a similar report, this time from
Uganda.[8] In the 1950s, before the discovery of HBV, it wasn't possible to test their hypothesis—that viral hepatitis was the cause of
HCC—directly. But this work could be undertaken after the tests
for Australia antigen became available. Professor Payet wanted to
collaborate with me on a study in Senegal to test the hypothesis.
Inspired by my recent experience in Uganda, I agreed to do so, and
this started what could be called the francophone phase of our research experience.

Beginning in 1974 I took part in a series of field trips to Senegal
and Mali, along with Tom London, William Wills (the entomologist),
and others from our laboratory in cooperation with a series of
young French physicians, mostly connected with the Institut de
Médecine et d'Épidémiologie Africaine at the Hôpital Claude Bernard, as well as Professor Payet and a number of Senegalese physicians. These included Bernard Larouze, Veronique Barrois, Lamine
Diakhate, Gerard Saimot, M. Sankale, Alain Froment, Evelyne Mari-
nier, Elisabeth Feret, A. Moustapha Sow, and others. We also com-
municated frequently, and occasionally collaborated, with Professor
Philippe Maupas and his colleagues at the University of Tours, a
very active group. A full account of the field and laboratory work,
of the comings and goings among Paris, Philadelphia, Dakar, Bamako, and places in between, would be a long, complex, and inter-

---

[7] M. Payet, R. Camain, and P. Pene, "Le cancer primitif du foie. Etude critique à
propos de 240 cas," *Revue Internationale d'Hepatologie* 4 (1956): 1–20.
[8] P. Steiner and J. N. Davies, "Cirrhosis and Primary Liver Carcinoma in Ugandan
Africans," *British Journal of Cancer* 11 (1957): 523–34.

esting saga, but there is no need to detail all of this here. After the projects were completed and our French and Senegalese colleagues had departed, our lives seemed less exciting and certainly less turbulent. There is a sequel. Tom London and his colleagues are still involved in a very large and long-term program with the armed forces of Senegal, studying primary cancer of the liver and its prevention.

To give some idea of the flavor of this period, I can recount an automobile trip Bernard Larouze and I took in Bamako (the capital of Mali) one dark tropical night. We were proceeding at speed on an unlighted main thoroughfare with many pedestrians, bicycles, horses, camels, and oxen sharing the way with us. The red dust was spewing about us, caught up in a swirl around our rattling Renault. I turned to Bernard, who was driving, and said, "I don't know about the state of the windscreen on your side of the car, but I can't see anything through mine." Unperturbed and without slackening speed, Bernard responded, "I can't see very much through my side either, but it doesn't matter since the brakes don't work." I should mention that, in addition to his ironic sense of humor, Bernard was an excellent scientific collaborator and a good friend.

Senegal and Mali produced interesting results. We found that there was a high frequency of antibody against the core (anti-HBc)—an indicator of viral replication—and that it was significantly different from what was seen in controls. This was confirmed in studies on patients from Hong Kong and Philadelphia. In a paper published in 1975,[9] we suggested that vaccination could prevent HCC. The recommendation was repeated in a paper published the following year reporting on our test of the hypothesis that mothers transmitted HBV to their children, who subsequently developed HCC. We identified patients with HCC and tested their parents and sibs for their responses to HBV infection and compared the results to those for control families (i.e., the families of parent controls who did *not* have

---

[9] P. Maupas, B. Larouze, W. T. London, B. Werner, I. Millman, A. O'Connell, B. S. Blumberg, G. Saimot, and M. Payet, "Antibody to Hepatitis-B Core Antigen in Patients with Primary Hepatic Carcinoma," *Lancet* 2 (1975): 9–11.

HCC). There was a much higher frequency of infection with HBV in the *mothers* but not the fathers of the HCC patients compared to the controls. Ed Lustbader executed another of his ingenious statistical analyses and estimated that the risk of HCC in the offspring of HBV carrier mothers was about five- to twelvefold, in the same range as the risk for cancer of the lung in cigarette smokers. In retrospect, this was, from a practical point of view, a very important study. We realized that much of the cancer in Africa—and, by extrapolation, elsewhere where mother-to-child transmission was common—could be prevented by infant immunization.

That raised a very important question. If the virus was transmitted from mothers to children before or at the moment of birth, would it be possible to vaccinate infants *prior* to their infection? We did a large study on maternal transmission, described in the next chapter, in Thies,[10] a provincial city east of Dakar. We concluded that, in Africa, transmission from the mother, although very common, does not occur until months or years after birth. This allows time for vaccination. By contrast, in many parts of Asia, transmission may occur before, at the moment of, or shortly after birth. But even in these locations there is an interval of a few weeks when vaccination is feasible before chronic infection sets in. These observations and more extensive ones by other scientists have established the importance of infant and early childhood vaccination. This has proven to be the mainstay of most of the national HBV immunization programs in regions where HBV is very common in the population.

There was another interesting observation that arose from Ed's analysis, unexpected when we started the study—a good example of new hypotheses arising when an initial hypothesis is being tested. The immune response of the fathers and sibs to infection, as measured by their development of anti-HBs, was less than in the fathers and sibs of controls who did not have HCC. We hypothesized that there was something else in the environment of these cancer families that diminished the immune response; we invoked

---

[10] Among other amenities of the place was "CAT" (Centre Amicale Thiessienne), a charming restaurant and bar not far from the study site.

aflatoxin,[11] a highly toxic material that is elaborated by fungi of the genus *Aspergillus*. These fungi can infest grains and other food-stuffs—for example, peanuts, which are widely grown and eaten in Senegal—that are improperly stored. (Aflatoxin had been suspected as a cause of cancer of the liver for many years, and there had been, and continues to be, extensive research programs in Africa and else-where to explore its role in the process.) Families with aflatoxin in their foodstuffs would be at greater risk for HCC. We know now that there is a strong synergistic carcinogenic effect of aflatoxin and HBV. Although the case for HBV as an etiologic and preventable cause of HCC was growing stronger, we wanted to understand, and emphasize, the interaction of many risk factors that increase the probability of cancer in the infected person.

Similar studies were being done in Asia, and we, in collaboration with several Korean colleagues, did a number of studies in Seoul, Korea. Dr. Hei-wan Hann, who worked in my laboratory for many years, was the central investigator in these studies.

Epidemiology in Taiwan

What to my mind was the most convincing epidemiolog-ical study on HBV as a cause of HCC was done by Professor Palmer Beasley, working in Taiwan. Tom London and I were asked to write a review on the important epidemiological studies on HBV.[12] We se-lected Palmer's study as one of these. Palmer and his Chinese col-leagues asked the question "Does the HBV carrier state precede the development of HCC?" They also wished to determine the inci-dence of HCC in HBV carriers, and to estimate the carriers' risk of getting HCC. They recruited 22,707 male government employees into the study between November 1975 and June 1978, and tested

---

[11] A genetic hypothesis is also tenable. The altered immune response in the fathers could be a consequence of a polymorphism with a specific immune effect, present in the fathers and inherited by their offspring. I will have more to say about this ap-proach in a later chapter.

[12] W. T. London and B. S. Blumberg, "Comments on the Role of Epidemiology in the Investigation of Hepatitis B Virus," *Epidemiologic Reviews* 7 (1985): 59–79.

all of them to identify carriers. The employees were covered by a single health insurance scheme, and information on cause of death could be obtained from their records. Anyone who developed HCC would also be reported to the insurance authorities. The study population was divided into two groups, HBsAg(+) and HBsAg(-). By the end of December 1980, 307 of the men had died, 41 from HCC. Of the HCC cases, 40 of the 42 developed in the HBV carriers. The incidence of HCC in the carriers was 351/100,000 population, compared to 55/100,000 for the entire population. On the basis of these initial data the relative risk for HCC was an astounding 223—that is, the carriers were more than two hundred times more likely to develop HCC than the men who were not carriers. These data also demonstrated the gravity of the problem: fully 13 percent (41 of 307 total deaths) of all the men in the cohort who had died, died from cancer of the liver. They were also at greatly increased risk for death from liver disease other than cancer. There were an additional 19 deaths due to cirrhosis of the liver, and 17 of these were carriers of HBV.

There have been several studies similar to these to determine risk to carriers in Alaska, China, and elsewhere. In general, the risk ratios were not as high (the Beasley risk estimates dropped in subsequent analysis also), but they were essentially all in the same direction. HBV is a great risk factor for HCC. It was no wonder that the health authorities in Taiwan gave HBV prevention top priority; as we shall see in the next chapter, they accelerated the vaccination program to very good effect.

These epidemiological studies made it highly likely that HBV was a cause of HCC. But there are other "causes" or factors that increase risk of a carrier's developing HCC, and in subsequent years many of these were identified. Hepatitis C virus (HCV) can cause cancer of the liver without apparent HBV infection, although sometimes there is also integration of HBV genomes in the cells of the cancer patients with HCV. Aflatoxins, smoking, alcohol, arsenic in water and food, and increased levels of iron stored in the body may all impose additional risk.

Fox Chase Cancer Center was funded mostly by the National Cancer Institute of the National Institutes of Health, and although there was a great deal of tolerance for research that did not involve cancer per se, there was a presumption that the funded research would sooner or later be relevant to cancer. (In Appendix 3, I comment on the research style of the NIH and how it influenced our research process.) When I joined FCCC in 1964, my research did not appear to have a rich cancer content. We were studying inherited biochemical and immunological diversity. Our first definitive paper on Australia antigen[13] did have a reference to the association of HBV with leukemia, but the argument was not strong. So even though the director of FCCC, Tim Talbot, with his typical intelligence, never pressed us to get on the cancer research track, we realized that it would be a good idea to show involvement, sooner rather than later. The connection between HBV and HCC, a very common cancer, that emerged from the trip to Uganda, along with the research we founded upon that connection, was a big step in the right direction.

Despite the impressive epidemiological evidence, scientists and the public lust after explanatory models, and molecular biology has supplied putative mechanisms to explain how HBV can cause cancer. It is to these that I turn in the following chapter.

---

[13] B. S. Blumberg, H. J. Alter, and S. Visnich, "A 'New' Antigen in Leukemia Sera," *Journal of the American Medical Association* 191 (1965): 541–46.

11. What Is Now Known about HBV?

IN THE PRECEDING CHAPTERS, I have recounted the early research that led to the discovery of HBV, the diagnostic techniques that improved the safety of the blood supply, the invention of the vaccine, and the causative relation of HBV to primary cancer of the liver. The major applications flowed directly from the rather primitive early discoveries before the techniques of molecular biology were well understood and applied. In this chapter, I will describe some of the research that followed the initial discovery that has added enormously to the understanding of HBV. This includes methods of transmission, epidemiology, the occurrence of viruses similar to HBV in other animals, the possible role of insects in transmission, the role of human gender, and the effects of the worldwide vaccination programs. Since the 1980s, research on the molecular biology of HBV has been undertaken brilliantly in many laboratories around the world. It has led to a much better understanding of the virus itself and to improved application, particularly of the vaccine. Perhaps of even greater importance, these developments point the direction for additional preventive measures for other cancers with a viral cause: those already known, as well as others that will be discovered in the future. The apparent success of HBV vaccination in preventing primary liver cancer provides a guide and builds confidence in the search for new methods of fighting and preventing cancer.

The virus has four genes (or open reading frames), designated *S* for the surface antigen protein, *C* for the protein that covers the inner core and encloses the DNA, P for the polymerase enzyme protein responsible for replication and other processes, and X for the X protein involved in transcription and, possibly, the carcinogenic properties of HBV. Additional details about the molecular biology of HBV are given in Appendix 4.

Transmission and Epidemiology of HBV

In the previous chapters, I have referred frequently to the epidemiology of HBV. In this section I will summarize the extensive information that is now available. Some of this emerged from our earliest studies on HBV, since so many of them were population-based, but most has come from the extensive studies by investigators all over the world.

HBV is very common in Asia and Africa, the parts of the world with the largest populations, as well as in other highly populated regions in eastern and central Europe and Central and South America. Amazingly, over half of the world's population have been infected or will become infected with HBV during the course of their lifetimes. (Most infections do not result in disease; the formation of protective anti-HBs is the most frequent outcome.) Over the centuries these two organisms, humans and HBV, have been intimate and interactive with each other. As with retroviruses like HIV, sequences of the HBV genome can integrate into the human genome and, in effect, become part of the human cell and body. It is not surprising that HBV is involved with some of the most critical events in the human life cycle. Attempting to treat chronic HBV infection confronts us with the Pogo paradox: "We have met the enemy and he is us."

There are three time periods in the life cycle of humans when transmission is most likely: (1) around the time of birth ("perinatal"), (2) early childhood, and (3) adulthood. The probability of an infected person's becoming a chronic carrier is strikingly age related. Newborns of mothers who are carriers with actively replicating HBV (they will usually have HBeAg in their blood) have an 85 percent or greater chance of becoming infected. If the carrier mother is HBeAg negative, the probability decreases to about 30 percent, but it is still much higher than for the newborns of mothers who are not HBV carriers. Older children, when infected, have a lower risk of becoming a carrier, and adults even less so. There is a fascinating geographic difference in the time and the character of the transmission. In the late 1970s and early 1980s we did an extensive series of studies in Senegal and Mali in collaboration with Senegalese and French colleagues to which I have already referred. Blood was collected from nearly fifteen hundred pregnant women attending the mother-child ("well baby") clinic in the provincial city of Thies. Their responses to HBV infection were recorded. At birth, blood was collected from the umbilical cord (which reflects the status in the child at and before birth); collections were repeated on several occasions for weeks or months afterward. In some cases, the collections went on for more than three years. As expected, children born to the mothers who were carriers of HBV—HBsAg(+)—had a much higher probability of becoming infected *and* of becoming carriers of HBV than children whose mothers were uninfected or who had anti-HBs. However, none of the children became infected before five months of age. This was in sharp contrast to the observations in Asia, where the children of carrier mothers nearly always became chronically infected within the first few weeks after birth. This meant that there was an interval after birth, longer in Senegal than in Asia, when the children were not chronically infected and could, theoretically, be vaccinated. The vaccine trials demonstrated that this was actually the case. The existence of this interval was, to use a somewhat unscientific term, providential. It meant that vaccination could be effective in newborns, preventing the development of chronic infection in exactly the age group that was otherwise most likely to become carriers. This biological characteristic of maternal transmission has permitted the extensive vaccination programs that have had such an impact on the epidemic of HBV, as I will describe later. It has nearly eliminated maternal-child transmission in the countries where the vaccination programs are effective.

One of the most gratifying experiences I have had as a scientist and physician was during a late-night dinner party in a cozy restaurant in Naples. My host, a colleague and international authority on hepatitis, told me that before the vaccine became available, he had had to counsel pregnant woman who were HBV carriers to consider abortion, since the likelihood of an infected child was so high. He now no longer had to do this, and he expressed his thanks to me, and to all those who had done research on hepatitis B, on behalf of the mothers of Italy. This was especially meaningful to Jean and me since our daughter-in-law, mother of two of our grandchildren, is herself from Naples.

The studies in Senegal and in many other locations enriched our understanding of what happens in early childhood. The probability of infection in young children during the first few months and years after birth is increased if mothers and, particularly, siblings are carriers. The means by which infection is transmitted are not entirely clear. The virus can be transmitted by breast-feeding, but in highly endemic areas other means of transmission would probably lead to infection whether or not the mother was breast-feeding. Before the vaccination programs were in place, in regions with poor childhood nutrition, breast-feeding was deemed to be more important than the possibility of HBV infection, and mothers were encouraged to continue the practice. In developed societies, as a precaution, HBV carrier mothers were encouraged not to breast-feed, since adequate nonmaternal food supplies were available. Of course, when vaccination is in place, breast-feeding is not a public health problem. Insects may also play a role in early childhood infection and will be discussed in greater detail below. It has been hard to determine how important insect transmission actually is. Possibly, with better control of other mechanisms of transmission, this question may assume greater importance. But, again, vaccination could render the problem of insect transmission moot. The general proximity of children to their mother and their sibs, the possibility of infection through open skin lesions, and the sharing of various personal and household implements probably account for the higher prevalence of infection in families where carriers are common. Paradoxically, we found that a carrier father in a family did not greatly increase risk. This probably results from fathers' interacting less with their children than mothers do, or than children do with one another—at least in the regions where the studies have been done—and reinforces the widely held maternal opinion that fathers don't spend enough time with the kids.

In young adults, the most common method of transmission is sexual. As might be expected, this risk decreases in the later decades of life when connubial couples find other interests. There is an increased risk of infection with an increasing number of partners for both homosexual and heterosexual contacts, and with the incidence of other venereal diseases. The open lesions in the venereal areas caused by syphilis, gonorrhea, and other sexually transmitted diseases may facilitate the transmission of HBV. Other blood-borne viruses may also be transmitted sexually. The public is familiar with the importance of sexual transmission of HIV; this information, widely disseminated by the media, has led to major changes in sexual attitudes, at least for a while, and is credited with blunting the full energy of the sexual revolution of the 1960s and 1970s. Although health authorities were well aware of the venereal spread of HBV, even before the beginning of the AIDS epidemic, this knowledge did not have much of an effect on public attitudes. This is probably because hepatitis was seen as a relatively benign disease from which recovery was the usual outcome. At that time, it was not widely appreciated that chronic infection, with its unhappy consequences, could also occur. The deadly character of HIV infection was much more effective as a deterrent, at least in some communities. HCV and human T cell-lymphotropic virus (HTLV) can also be transmitted sexually. The risk of sexual transmission is greater for HBV than the others under most circumstances.

Ritual practices, such as tattooing, provide another mechanism of transmission in older children and adults. Tattooing has probably been a significant factor in the spread of HBV in indigenous societies where major segments of the population are ritually tattooed, often in large group events. It has also had an effect in more developed countries. In the 1970s and earlier, tattooing parlors had a limited clientele, such as itinerant sailors and other defined social groups. I can dimly recall a personal near-tattooing experience when, as a teenage sailor, I was a member of a recreational party whose concluding event was to be a mass tattooing. I had already selected the motif for my decoration (was it "Death Before Dishonor" superim-

posed on a dagger entering a stylized heart, or simply "Mother"?),
but when the chips were down, my homeboy values surfaced, and
I opted out amid universal expressions of disgust. In recent decades
tattooing has become far more common and more sophisticated. In
the pre-HBV discovery period, the needles used for the process were
sometimes used on successive clients, usually without the rigorous
cleaning required for eliminating HBV. When the testing capabilities
for HBV became available, the public health authorities could
clearly demonstrate that needle puncture was a mechanism of transmission, and laws were passed in many jurisdictions requiring the
use of disposable needles. This has saved many from the misery of
acute or chronic HBV infection.

There are a surprisingly large number of other ritual practices by
which blood, and blood-borne viruses, can be spread from one individual to another. A student in my medical anthropology class once
compiled a list of the practices, with pictures, for her term paper. It
included cicatrix formation on the skin,[1] ritual circumcision,[2] acu-
puncture, "blood brothers" and "blood sisters,"[3] needle sharing
among intravenous drug addicts, and others. Vaccination would obviously decrease the risk inherent in these practices. It is not clear how
often they contribute to the overall risk of HBV infection, but transmission of hepatitis among illegal drug users is one of the most common causes of acute and chronic HBV hepatitis in the United States.

It also is one of the major routes for the transmission of HCV and
HIV. Since the 1980s I have, on several occasions, been consulted by
patients, physicians, and family members concerning cases of chronic

---

[1] A technique of scarring the skin in a series of points forming a desired pattern
that becomes apparent following the formation of scar tissue or keloid. It was widely
used in Nigeria during the period of my field trip in 1957. Often the same instrument
was used on many people.

[2] In many cultures mass circumcision involving a number of children might be
done at the time that a group of them entered a certain age range. One person after
the next would be cut with the same circumcision device without adequate cleaning
between uses.

[3] A large percentage of one of my medical anthropology classes at the University
of Pennsylvania claimed that they had established a blood sibship with friends or
actual sibs by piercing their fingers and intermixing blood. This appears to have been
a frequent blood exchange folk practice in Western urban and suburban society.

hepatitis due to HBV and/or HCV, which were a result of intravenous drug use during the patient's youth in the drug-happy 1960s and 1970s. The stories were poignant and tragic; the patients were often successful citizens, happily ensconced in the suburbs with their wives and children, enjoying a respectable middle-class life. They learned that they were carriers, and probably had been for decades, when they had a routine blood test or as a consequence of what they considered to be minor symptoms. It is a terrible irony that the consequences of these apparently trivial adventures of a carefree and liberated youth should persist to torment their middle years.

In the late 1960s we collaborated with scientists at the U.S. Army Medical Research Laboratory at Fort Knox, Kentucky, in a study of more than sixteen hundred members of the Armored Brigade; the cohort included both soldiers who had recently returned from Vietnam and recruits who had not yet been to southeast Asia. There was a significantly higher frequency of HBV carriers among the returnees (about 0.7 percent)[4] than among the recruits (0.2 percent). In the early 1970s we did a second and larger study involving nearly twenty thousand Vietnam War returnees and recruits. We also had data on returnees who were participating in a drug rehabilitation program. Our conclusion was that essentially all the increase in the number of carriers among the returnees could be accounted for by the much higher prevalence of carriers (2.5 percent) among the drug users. Although the total number of carriers who returned to the States was high, the percentage of soldiers who became carriers was low—less than 1 percent. Many more must have been exposed, developed anti-HBs with or without acute hepatitis, and recovered. In fact, acute hepatitis was one of the main causes of illness in the military in Vietnam, and a significant part of this was probably a consequence of needle use.

There are bizarre mechanisms of transmission that illustrate how clever HBV can be in finding victims to perpetuate itself in the human population. Orienteering is a popular sport in Sweden, as it

---

[4] These studies were done with the very insensitive immunodiffusion method for detecting HBsAg. If the radioimmunoassay had been available, the prevalence would have been found to be much higher.

is in many European and other countries. It consists of running from point to point in the forests and fields, armed with map and compass in an effort to reach all the control points without getting lost and to arrive at the end point ahead of competitors. It is a healthy out-of-doors sport undertaken by fit and athletic people, young and old. In the 1970s there was a report of an epidemic of hepatitis B infection involving several hundred orienteers. How did this happen? An epidemiological investigation revealed the probable cause. At the time, the athletes usually ran through the brush wearing shorts. They would sustain multiple minor lacerations and abrasions from the undergrowth. At some of the control stations, buckets of water and towels were provided to clean the bloody legs. Also, small drops of blood would remain on the vegetation on the commonly used tracks. Hepatitis B carriers are rare in Scandinavian populations, but apparently there were a sufficient number to contaminate the wash water and/or the vegetation. The solution to the problem? As is often the case in preventive medicine, if the mechanism of transmission is known, remedial solutions are obvious. Orienteers now wear leg coverings when they run through the woods.

There is another tale that can be construed as the adaptation of HBV to a major change in human behavior—the use of computers. In the 1970s a report appeared on the transmission of HBV in a hospital that had recently installed a computer-based system for the recording and transfer of laboratory data.[5] In those bygone times (at least on the computer timescale), IBM punch cards were used to record data for input into the computer. The hospital system involved moving the punched card from the clinic to the laboratory and other parts of the hospital. Those of you old enough to remember the then ubiquitous punch cards (I recall a ticker-tape parade on lower Broadway in New York City that included showers of them) will know that it was easy to sustain a thin laceration from their sharp edges. Apparently, such cuts had been sufficient to allow transmission of the virus from cards on which contaminated blood speci-

---

[5] C. P. Pattison, D. M. Boyer, J. E. Maynard, and P. C. Kelly, "Epidemic Hepatitis in a Clinical Laboratory: Possible Association with Computer Card Handling," *Journal of the American Medical Association* 230 (6) (1974): 854–57.

mens had been spilled to several people who had contact with the card. Another remarkable example of adaptation! Obviously, an organism with only four genes doesn't plan strategy—but ponder for a moment the "cleverness" of these schemes to adapt to a human behavior to ensure infection.

Under natural conditions, before the introduction of needles and skin-piercing medical devices, the rise of the drug culture, and other human behaviors that can result in blood-borne transmission, the main methods of spread would have been, as noted above, mother-to-child transmission, sexual transmission, and transmission within households. HBV has managed to insinuate itself into the main functions that allow humans to perpetuate themselves: childbirth, sexual union, and family interaction. The replication activities of the virus are such that it can maintain relatively high levels of infectious virus in the bloodstream of the infected during the periods when its host is occupied with these human species–maintaining functions. Although infection may occur at the moment of birth, or even before, death from HBV infection occurs many years later in the fourth, fifth, and later decades of life when the HBV carrier may develop chronic liver disease and primary hepatocellular carcinoma. It doesn't kill its host until the later decades of life when the possibilities of transmission are greatly decreased. It is as if the virus acts as a symbiote as long as the humans serve its goals of transmission, and then hastens the death of its "companion" humans when they are no longer of use.

But is it a true symbiosis? Are there any advantages that accrue to the human host? Polymorphic traits have advantages and disadvantages; since we had reason to believe the HBV carrier state was polymorphic (i.e., that the genes for and resistance to chronic infection that we hypothesized were polymorphisms), there might be some advantage to the carrier state. Maybe. I will describe what may be an example of an advantage.

For several years we studied the relation of the amount of iron stored in the body to the development and retention of the carrier state, the replication of HBV in the host, and the pathogenesis of chronic liver disease and hepatocellular carcinoma. We found that the levels of the proteins used for the storage of iron were signifi-

cantly higher in the carriers of HBV than in those who had responded to infection by producing anti-HBs, or who had not been
infected. To put it differently, carriers retained more iron from their
diet than did noncarriers. This could be an advantage in regions
where diet iron is low, particularly in the young, who require iron
to optimize their metabolism and for the production of hemoglobin.
It would also be an advantage to women of childbearing age, who,
even in regions where the diet is optimal, require supplemental iron
during pregnancy and often at other times as well.[6] The disadvantages of the carrier state would only be manifest decades later when
the host developed chronic liver disease and/or cancer of the liver.
However, in premodern times life expectancy would not have extended beyond the first few decades of life, and HBV carriers would
die from other causes before the late detrimental effects of HBV infection kicked in.

There are probably other effects of the HBV carrier state that are
advantageous. For example, the increased prevalence of male children, which, as we will discuss below, occurs in the families of HBV
carriers, might be construed as an advantage in some societies. But,
as you might imagine, there has been little research on the benefits
accrued to HBV carriers; viruses are not usually regarded as being
of any value to their human hosts.

Hepadna Viruses in Other Animals

The discovery of HBV viruses in animals other than humans has been important not only from the standpoint of studying
the coevolution of animals and the viruses that infect them, but also

---

[6] We did many studies on the iron-binding proteins that store and transport iron in
the body, but time and space preclude my describing these in detail. Our conclusion,
consistent with a great deal of research conducted by others, was that increased iron
stores helped to perpetuate the carrier state and increased the risk of chronic liver
disease and cancer of the liver. Richard Stevens, an epidemiology graduate student
who worked in my laboratory for many years (and was also my running guru), did
much of this research as part of his doctoral thesis. He found that increased body
storage iron imposed an increased risk for many kinds of cancer, a fascinating finding
with many implications for the prevention and treatment of cancer.

in working out the replication process for the whole family of viruses. In addition, it could be of value in the diagnosis and eventual treatment of disease in the animals themselves.

The actual discovery of new species of HBV-like viruses in other animal species came about in the unpredictable, serendipitous manner that characterizes research. I will tell you the story as far as I am aware of it.

A local drug company gave us a gibbon that had been infected with HBV. They were concerned about retaining an animal that might infect the handlers and others; they thought that we could utilize it for observation and research. To ensure proper care, we arranged to have it admitted to the Philadelphia Zoological Garden, the oldest zoo in America—Philadelphia is filled with "the oldest" of all kinds—where it was placed under the care of Dr. Robert Snyder, the director of research. We did not experiment on the animal but did observe it carefully for any signs of disease and obtained biological specimens from time to time for laboratory study. During our occasional visits we often spoke with Robert, and at some point we mentioned our interest in cancer of the liver. He responded something to the effect that if we were interested in cancer of the liver, we had come to the right place. He had been studying woodchucks (*Marmota monax*, also known as groundhogs) for many years and had done his doctoral thesis on aspects of their sex ratio. Much of his fieldwork had been done at the Letterkenny Arsenal in central Pennsylvania, a vast acreage used, in part, for the storage of military equipment and supplies. Ammunition was stored in huge underground magazines. Woodchucks were a problem because they burrowed into the earth-covered mounds and compromised safe storage. The military was interested in thoroughly understanding the biology of these active animals. Woodchucks are also a major agricultural problem in many parts of the eastern United States.

Robert had retained a sizable number of animals in suitable enclosures at the zoo and, over the course of the years, had discovered that as many as 30 percent of them died of primary cancer of the liver. When he looked for liver cancer in animals that had been captured in the wild, the numbers were much lower. Wild woodchucks apparently don't live as long as animals kept in the salubrious environment of the Philadelphia Zoo. If corrections were made for the much lower age of death of the wild-living animals, then they too were seen to have a very high prevalence of liver cancer.

At about this time, Jesse Summers, a virologist at Fox Chase Cancer Center who had been working on other viruses, expressed an interest on working on HBV. He was looking for an animal in which it would be more feasible to study replication (for some reason, possibly because he is an avid fisherman, he wanted to study fish), and Tom London suggested that he look at the *Marmota*. We had already tried to find evidence of HBV infection using the specific antibody against HBsAg but had been unsuccessful. Jesse, using recently available molecular biology methods, was able to identify a virus and eventually see it in an electron microscope; it was named woodchuck hepatitis virus (WHV). Bill Mason, also at FCCC, and Jesse then began the research that, in time, led to an understanding of the replication cycle of this whole family of viruses.

The discovery of a related virus in another species spurred a search for additional examples. Another chance experience was associated with the discovery of the second nonhuman HBV-like virus. In the mid-1970s, an abstract was submitted to an international cancer congress by scientists from the People's Republic of China, describing an extensive study on primary cancer of the liver involving thousands of cases. It was evident from the numbers given in the paper that liver cancer was a major problem in China, afflicting far more patients than were stricken, to our knowledge, anywhere else in the world. The vaccine and the results of all the recent research on HBV would find its greatest application in that vast country, which even then had a population probably exceeding one billion. This was before the United States had established diplomatic relations with China, and Western visitors were rare. I wrote to the medical authorities, expressing my interest in traveling to China to discuss the recent advances in the field and, in particular, the vaccine. I got a reply but no further encouragement. However, shortly after I was awarded the Nobel Prize in 1976, I received an invitation from the Chinese Medical Association—which, I was assured, was a nongovernmental organization[7]— to visit and to speak

---

[7] I believe that this was because the United States and the People's Republic of China had not yet established formal diplomatic relations with one another. The invi-

to scientists. The trip itself, in October 1977, soon after the unseating of the Gang of Four and before the opening of the country to Western influence and trade, was fascinating, but I will spare you another travelogue. I visited major cities and spoke to thousands of scientists. I was accompanied for a large portion of the trip by Dr. T.-T. Sun, a senior scientist who, before the Cultural Revolution, had been working in theoretical biophysics. During the revolution he had been sent to practice medicine in the countryside in Kweilin Autonomous Region and became aware of the importance of hepatocellular carcinoma. He was a national and later an internationally recognized expert on hepatitis who has made important contributions to the field. The other member of our party, Mr. Lee, was a guide provided by the Chinese Medical Association. He had been a Red Guard.

We had ample opportunity to talk during long walks we took in the evening after my schedule of lectures. He told me that in the regions of China where cancer of the liver was common in humans, it was also common in domestic ducks. An interesting observation, typical of the anecdotal items that often turn into important research. Blood samples from Chinese ducks from Chi-tung County (on the north bank of the Yangtze River across from Shanghai) were sent to my laboratory and given to Jesse Summers and Bill Mason, the scientists who had worked on the woodchuck virus. A virus similar in appearance to HBV was seen in eleven of the thirty-three duck bloods we received. During the course of their studies they were inoculating domestic U.S. ducks ("Pekin" ducks, a popular American breed derived originally from Chinese stock) and found that the uninoculated "control" ducks contained an HBV-like virus! The duck virus, named duck hepatitis B virus (DHBV), was present in high prevalence in many duck flocks in the United States. The duck model has been used widely in the study of replication and pathogenesis of the whole class of Hepadna viruses. Dr. Sun, independently, identified a similar virus in the Chinese ducks.

---

tation, therefore, was from a private organization to a private citizen. However, when I was in China, all my contacts seemed to be at a governmental or party level. I was usually greeted at the airport by a junior minister and the secretary of the Communist Party cadre and provided with a politically knowledgeable guide and translator from a government agency.

When I think back to the trip, it is the tranquil moments in a very hectic program that I remember best. I was with fellow Chinese scientists or Party and government officials most of the time, but no one seemed to mind what I did when I was by myself. I would arise early in the morning and run five or six miles in whatever city or rural location we had spent the night in. In Beijing, the streets would be mostly empty, but in small parks and alleys bands of people, young and old, would be going through their tai chi exercises quietly and in unison. Near Kweilin, I ran for miles along a riverside path going through farmyards and intensely cultivated fields, among farmers walking and riding out to the fields from the collective's buildings. People were too polite to stare at me, even though an awkward Western runner could not have been a common sight. I recall a Sunday when we were not working and Dr. Sun and Mr. Lee took me to a teahouse in a pleasant grove of trees with magnificent bamboos partially shielding the view of a sparkling mountain stream. The conversation was in Chinese, with occasional outbursts of laughter; Dr. Sun or Mr. Lee would translate a brief synopsis of the lead-in and a detailed explication of the punch line. But most of the time I was content to sit and hear the rhythmic flow of conversation, a member of the group, but pleasantly separated from it, listening to my own thoughts.

The end of October was cold in Beijing, with bitter winds sweeping in from Siberia. I had bought an immense padded cotton coat, and in the evenings, capped by a proportionately large woolen cap, I would walk the streets alone in the midst of a vast crowd of pedestrians and cyclists, stopping at a communal kitchen or a teahouse from time to time, soaking in the sense of the enormous city.

The trip to the People's Republic of China was one of the most important, if not the most important foreign excursion I have ever undertaken in respect to the impact that it had on the public health. I reported on the latest research on hepatitis and its application to audiences who knew little of it, and even carried information from one laboratory in China to another. I told them about our HBV vaccine, provided a copy of the patent (which had already been published), and set up for contacts with Merck, with whom we had signed our patent licensing agreement. Arrangements were made later by Merck and the Chinese authorities for technology transfer that allowed the construction of facilities for the manufacture of the vaccine. In later years, visiting Chinese scientists would often tell me that they had heard me speak, and of the effect my visit had on accelerating research and initiating the huge vaccination program that is now in place.

The vaccination program in China is, possibly, the largest in the world. However, the full potential of the vaccination program has not been realized, in part because of the high cost of the vaccine. In addition, as noted in the *New York Times* (20 August 2001), the Chinese health authorities are concerned about the transmission of HBV through needle injection. Frequent injection of antibiotics and other medications is common in local medical practice, particularly in children. Disposable needles and syringes are often reused, often without adequate cleaning, because of their high cost. This has greatly increased the possibility of transmission and the prevalence of infection, particularly in the young, who are more prone to become carriers when infected. It would be advantageous if means could be found to distribute the vaccine more widely to effect universal vaccination in the country that, probably, has the largest number of HBV carriers in the world.

To return to our Stateside research trajectory—we had requested supplemental funding from our granting agency to search for additional animal viruses, but they deemed this a lower priority than other investigations, and our request was denied. They reckoned that there were already sufficient animal models and any further information would be redundant. I, of course, felt differently and argued that a study of the natural history and the evolutionary relations between the animals and the viruses that infected them, independent of any immediate application, would broaden understanding. There is a school of thought in research funding which seeks to identify projects that have a high likelihood of hitting "pay dirt," either theoretical or applied. This is an approach that is hard to dispute—except by the argument that it works against the discovery of totally new ideas, ideas that cannot be anticipated on the basis of current knowledge.

Despite our setback, the search for additional viruses continued. Patricia Marion, an investigator at Stanford University Medical School, found an HBV-like virus in *Spermophilus beecheyii*, the dusky ground squirrel often seen rustling through the fallen leaves and boughs of the gum trees that are common in the wilder parts of that enormous campus. She retained the animals that carried the virus—which she designated ground squirrel hepatitis virus (GSHV)—for several years and discovered that a significant number of the carriers developed primary cancer of the liver. Related viruses have been found in several species of wild ducks, in herons (HHBV), geese, and, probably, tree squirrels (TSHBV).

Unexpectedly, the duck virus has proven to be very useful in the study of replication and in pathology studies. The virus is common (10 percent) in domestic flocks of ducks. It is transmitted in nature primarily from mothers to their fetuses. This induces an immune tolerance, and the ducks do not, as a rule, develop liver disease later in life. Also, antibodies are less likely to form, and it is easier to identify and study the intermediates in the replication cycle.

The viruses have a unique form of replication; strangely, there is a close similarity to the replication of the DNA plant virus Cauliflower Mosaic Virus! Think of the interesting evolutionary implications of that observation. There are two circular strands of DNA in HBV, but each has a gap in it—one large and the other small—so that, in effect, they are linear. There is a piece of protein bound to one end of the longer ("full-length") strand. After the virus enters the liver cell, the outer coating is removed and a full-length strand of RNA is transcribed[8] from the full-length DNA. The RNA strand, referred to as the "pre-genome" of the virus, is then covered with the core protein to form a small particle along with a virus-derived reverse transcriptase and a small piece of protein to serve as a primer. Then, within the core particle a strand of DNA is synthesized by the reverse transcription process, and the pre-genome is degraded and removed. In this respect HBV is similar to retroviruses (e.g., HIV), but in other aspects of its biology it is clearly distinct from them. The first DNA strand synthesizes the second incomplete strand of DNA. The core particle is then enveloped by the surface antigen, probably added at one of the small organs in the

---

[8] Transcription is the synthesis of RNA from the DNA template. This process was part of the initial "dogma."

cell (the reticuloendothelium system), sugars are added to the HBsAg, and the virus is ready for export from the cell to do its mischief elsewhere. The DNA of HBV can integrate into the host DNA, but this is not required for the replication of the virus.

The characteristics of the viruses were so unprecedented that the systematists decided it should constitute a new family of viruses, the *Hepadnaviridae*, that is, DNA viruses that have a tropism for the liver. There is close homology[9] among the mammalian viruses (*Orthohepadnaviridae*) and among the avian viruses (*Avihepadnaviridae*). Homology between HBV and WHV is greater than 70 percent, and between GSHV and HBV about 55 percent. WHV and GSHV have 82 percent homology. The homologies between the avian viruses and the mammalian viruses are much less extensive. WHV has other similarities to HBV, in that it causes chronic liver disease and primary cancer of the liver and has a similar, but not identical, method of pathogenesis and replication. It is, to my knowledge, one of the closest models between human disease and disease in another species that can be used for the study of the human disease as well as the animal disease. It is for this reason that, despite the difficulty in raising and caring for woodchucks, they have been used extensively in basic research and in the testing of drugs of potential value for the treatment of HBV.

Much of the success with the woodchucks is due to the work of Professor Bud C. Tennant of Cornell University School of Veterinary Medicine, who has established a breeding facility for these animals. He and his colleagues have performed some of the seminal studies on the relation of the *Hepadnaviridae* to primary cancer of the liver. They inoculated 43 woodchucks, raised in his breeding facility, at birth, and another 43 animals at eight weeks of age. Thirteen of the animals that were inoculated at birth (32 percent) became chronic carriers of WHV, while 28 cleared the infection and did not become carriers. (Two of the animals died early in the course of the study and could not be evaluated.) After three years of observation, 11 of the animals that had become chronically infected developed HCC;

---

[9] Homology is a measure of the similarity of the sequences of the different viruses' DNA.

of the 28 that had been transiently infected, two developed HCC. The outcomes were different in the animals inoculated at eight weeks. Twenty-three developed acute infection with WHV but only three became chronic carriers. Two of the three chronic carriers were followed for three years, and they both developed HCC. None of eight animals in this group who had incurred transient infections developed cancer. A control group of 46 animals that had *not* been inoculated were also followed for three years; none of them developed HCC. John Gerin extended these studies on animals at the facility at Cornell. A larger group of experimentally infected animals were followed for three years; 61 of 63 (97 percent) of chronic carriers of WHV and 11 of 63 (17 percent) transiently infected animals developed HCC. None of the 108 uninfected controls, followed for the same period of time, developed HCC.

A remarkable set of results. It represents a direct experimental demonstration of the role of WHV in the etiology of primary cancer of the liver and, because of the similarity of the viruses and the disease, by analogy, the role of HBV in the etiology of HCC in humans. It also demonstrates that infection soon after birth greatly increases the risk of becoming a carrier of WHV and, therefore, the risk of developing HCC. An unexpected finding in the woodchucks was that some of the animals that were transiently infected eventually developed HCC, although the risk was much less than for the carriers. There has been an assumption that acute hepatitis in humans does not result in cancer of the liver—that, rather, chronic infection with HBV is required. The whole set of studies was one of the most convincing experimental proofs that cancer can be caused by a virus. It should be pointed out that the molecular biology of primary liver cancer in woodchucks differs from that in humans. The HBV DNA does not regularly integrate adjacent to oncogenes or antioncogenes in humans. However, in about half of the liver cancer cases in woodchucks, the WHV sequences integrate adjacent to the N-*myc2* gene, a very well studied oncogene. This may account for the extraordinary carcinogenicity of WHV in its host. This *myc* integration isn't seen with the ground squirrel virus, where there is very much less cancer. Other proteins produced by the virus may also have a role in the carcinogenic process.

It has been fascinating watching the unfolding of the story of the Hepadna viruses in other species. In what species did the virus start? Was it transmitted from one species to the next, and if so, how? Or were there independent origins? Are there similar viruses in other species that have not yet been identified for lack of research funding to systematically advance the program? One can see the grand workings of the interactions between the different viruses and their hosts, widely separated in a direct evolutionary sense, but proximate to one another in the environments they share. There has been a mysterious dance, over the millennia, as the viruses and their hosts interacted with one another and, presumably, with other agents. It recalls the often-quoted "tangled bank" metaphor Charles Darwin coined in the concluding part of *The Origin of Species*.

It is interesting to contemplate a tangled bank, clothed with many plants of many kinds, with birds singing on the bushes, with various insects flitting about, and with worms crawling through the damp earth, and to reflect that these elaborately constructed forms, so different from each other, and dependent upon each other in so complex a manner, have all been produced by laws acting around us. These laws, taken in the largest sense, being Growth with Reproduction; Inheritance which is almost implied by reproduction; Variability from the indirect and direct action of the conditions of life, and from use and disuse: a Ratio of Increase so high as to load to a Struggle for Life, and as a consequence to Natural Selection, entailing Divergence of Character, and Extinction of less improved forms. Thus, from the war of nature, from famine and death, the most exalted object which we are capable of conceiving, namely, the production of the higher animals, directly follows. There is grandeur in this view of life, with its several powers, having been originally breathed by the Creator into a few forms or into one; and that, whilst this planet has gone on cycling on according to the fixed law of gravity, from so simple a beginning endless forms most beautiful and most wonderful have been, and are being evolved.[10]

[10] C. Darwin, *The Origin of Species* (New York: Random House, 1993), 648. I am grateful to J. N. Gardner, who invoked this image in his discussion of complexity in biology. (J. N. Gardner, "The Selfish Biocosm," *Complexity* 5 [2000]: 34–45.)

Can the other-than-human viruses cross the species boundary and infect humans? There is no evidence that this is the case, although there have been few epidemiological studies. Cross-species infection may occur; woodchucks have been infected with GSHV. At the moment, there seems to be little public health concern about human contacts with these animals. The history of medicine teaches that environments and interactions change, and animal-to-man transmission may occur if there are peculiar and unpredictable changes in behaviors and relationships. Obviously, more knowledge of the nonhuman viruses would help us prepare for and possibly prevent cross-species infections that might occur in the future.

Insects

Why did I become interested in insect transmission of HBV? This line of inquiry probably arose from my experience in tropical medicine. In the tropics human illness can be attributed to two main problems: human fecal contamination of water and food, and the transmission of disease-causing agents by various insects, mostly mosquitoes. It is notewothy that Alfred Prince, who has been one of the few scientists in the hepatitis field to pursue the question of insect transmission, has spent many years working in the tropics, primarily in West Africa. There are other reasons for my interest. Many viruses are spread by mosquitoes, insects are common transmitters of disease in the regions of the world where HBV is common, and, most important, insect spread can be controlled—although not easily.

The first mosquito collections were done during my visit to Uganda, where I conducted night collections in the game parks adjacent to settled communities. It was an anxiety-provoking exercise. The game wardens cautioned me not to wander around in the dark or in the early dawn when the hippopotamuses were finding their way to and from the river. Apparently lions and other predators were also active at night. The small batteries I had to power the light that attracted the insects, and to drive the fan that kept the mosquitoes in the trap, lasted only about ten hours. If the battery failed, the air draft would stop and the mosquitoes could escape. Just before dark, I would rush into the bush, affix the traps to trees adjacent to the village houses, and scamper back before the last rays of the sun disappeared. In the morning, after a sleepless night, I would scamper out, trying to smell and hear the animals that might be prowling about, and retrieve the bugs. They were then frozen and shipped out as soon as I could find transportation for them. There were also a few collections in Ethiopia.

There was a high prevalence of HBV detected in the mosquitoes, with field infection rates in some species of mosquito as high as 1:100. Later, Bill Wills,[11] the medical entomologist of the Commonwealth of Pennsylvania, collected mosquitoes in Senegal and again found a very high field infection rate. Bill and others also found a high prevalence of infected mosquitoes in other parts of the tropical and temperate world. Researchers could infect the mosquitoes experimentally by feeding them on the blood of a HBV carrier.

I decided that working with mosquitoes had its disadvantages when I noticed that even in an insectarium with multiple safeguards to retain the mosquitoes within their screened cages, there were still a few stray insects flying in the surrounding room. It didn't take a great stretch of the imagination to realize that this was an unfortunate feature of an experimental system in which the mosquitoes might be infected with HBV. We therefore looked at other insects—specifically, bedbugs. Studies were done in Senegal by Bill Wills and in Sabah (Malaysia) by Walter Ogston.[12] Walter and the others found that 60 percent of the tropical bedbugs (*Cimex hemipterus*) collected

---

[11] Bill subsequently came to work on the medical entomology of HBV in my laboratory. He was a good colleague and a good friend. As a young man he had fought during the Korean conflict and was caught in the retreat from the Chosin Reservoir when the Chinese army joined with the North Koreans and launched a massive winter attack on the United Nations forces. Following his discharge he returned to the United States and enrolled, as he told me, at the college at the farthest location to which his bus fare would take him. That turned out to be Chico State University in California, where he earned his degree in entomology.

[12] Walter is the son of Alexander Ogston, who was the supervisor for my graduate degree in Oxford. He was trained in ecology at Princeton University and came to work with us on insects. He subsequently did pioneering research on the molecular biology of HBV in Summer's laboratory.

from beds in Senegal whose main occupants were HBV carriers had the virus in their bodies. This was the highest field infection rate for any insect that we were aware of. After a meal of blood taken from an HBV carrier, bedbugs had HBV in their bodies for weeks and in their fecal matter for weeks after it had disappeared from the body parts. This raised the possibility that bedbug transmission could provide a mechanism for transfer of infection from one occupant of a bed to another. Transmission could be by bites from the same insect, or by ingestion or inhalation of the fecal dust present in the beds, a nonvenereal (and unromantic) form of connubial transmission. It could also account for transmission from mothers to their newborn infants with whom they shared a bed.

Despite these experimental possibilities, there has never been any solid evidence that bedbugs make a major contribution to the transmission of HBV. Andrew Hall, now at the London School of Tropical Medicine, was involved in a massive epidemiologic study in The Gambia, West Africa, on hepatitis B and the effect of vaccination on the prevention of HCC. He and his colleagues, in 1994, reported an interesting and well-done study. They identified several villages where the prevalence of HBV carriers was very high. People were selected who had not yet been infected with HBV and were divided into two groups. The beds of one group were treated systematically to eliminate bedbugs, and the other group's beds did not receive any treatment. The researchers examined the people over the next two years to compare the incidence of HBV infection between the two groups. There was about a 17 percent higher frequency in the nontreated group, but the difference was not statistically significant. Andy concluded that if there was an effect of bedbug transmission, it was not very large. It is still possible that bedbug transmission is fairly efficient, but that other methods of transmission are so effective that they conceal the bedbug effect. Epidemiology is supposed to tell us what is actually happening, while experimental studies tell us what *could* happen. For the moment, the excitement about insect transmission is muted.

Not surprisingly, we were unable to convince the granting authorities to fund more sophisticated studies—for example, to determine whether HBV replicated in insects. One of the few agencies funding medical entomology was the Department of Defense. They were interested in the mosquito-borne viruses that were common in tropical and Asian regions where the Army was active, or where they thought they might be in the future. They may also have had an interest in protection against the possible use of insect vectors to spread biological warfare agents. However, we did not pursue the project much further; and despite the apparent probability that insect transmission could occur, there has not been any convincing epidemiological evidence that it is an important factor in the spread of HBV disease. I still think it an intriguing problem, involving, as it does, complex biological systems interacting with one another. For example, HBV DNA integrates into the genome of infected human hosts. Could insects transmitting HBV carry with them small segments of the hosts' DNA sequences? Could insects act as a mechanism to transfer genetic material from one human to another, without sexual reproduction, and thus have an effect on the evolutionary history of the species they bite? Granted, conjectural, but conjecture is part of the fun of science.

The research on HBV and insects did have an odd, but important, application in quite an unexpected manner. In the early 1980s the public was very concerned with the alarming growth of the AIDS epidemic. The report of a very high incidence of AIDS in the community of Belle Glade in West Palm Beach County, Florida,[13] generated wide media attention. According to the initial observations, the cases could not be accounted for by the usual risk factors for AIDS transmission—venereal, mother to child, drug abuse, and the like. By default, the extraordinarily high prevalence was attributed to mosquitoes, which were very common in this region. This caused great alarm among public health officials, AIDS activists groups, and the government. If mosquitoes could transmit the HIV virus, then the whole social environment for patients with AIDS and carriers of HIV would become even more precarious. Insect transmission, if it occurred, meant that people within mosquito-flying range

[13] K. G. Castro, S. Lieb, H. W. Jaffe, J. P. Narkunas, C. H. Calisher, T. J. Bush, and J. J. Witte, "Transmission of HIV in Belle Glade, Florida: Lessons for Other Communities in the United States," *Science* 239 (1988): 193–97.

of a carrier would be at risk for HIV infection. The fear generated by this possibility could have resulted in a popular demand to remove HIV-infected people from the community. To investigate the issues raised in Belle Glade, the U.S. Congressional Office for Technical Assistance, a body set up to advise Congress on medical and scientific matters, decided to review the whole problem at a meeting convened in Washington, D.C.

Because of the similarities between the epidemiology and virology of HIV and HBV, I was asked to review the data on the possibility of insect transmission of HBV. We had substantial evidence that HBV *could* be transmitted by insects, even though there was not any proof of actual transmission in nature. On the other hand, there were few or no data supporting insect transmission of HIV. It was a heated and animated session, since some passionately believed that insects were responsible for transmission, and that this could be a more widespread problem. The conclusion of the conference was that HIV was not insect-transmitted, and this relieved a great deal of anxiety.

HBV and Gender

It is, I admit, hard to imagine that HBV is gender-biased. Of course, it isn't. How could an organism with only four genes conceive of bias? However, on the face of it, it appears to behave differently in its interactions with males and females, in some respects favoring women, and in others not. In the earliest epidemiologic studies we saw a higher prevalence of HBV carriers in males than in females in nearly all populations. We also found that, when infected, females were more likely than males to develop antibody against the surface antigen (the protective anti-HBs), and males more likely than females to become carriers of HBV (HBsAg). The ratio of males to females is higher in patients with chronic liver disease and in primary cancer of the liver, where it may be 7 or 8 to 1, or even higher.

Perhaps the strangest observation concerns the relation between the response of a parent to infection with HBV and the gender of his or her offspring. Let me run the data by you, but with the caution that most of these studies are from our laboratory, and there has not been very much confirmation of our results. Perhaps this is because virologists don't usually think that viruses have an effect on human gender, which, I must admit, is not an unreasonable view.

The first observations were made in a small provincial town in northern Greece that we had elected to study because of its high prevalence of hepatitis carriers. Much of the fieldwork and analysis were done by Jana Hesser, then a graduate student in anthropology at the University of Pennsylvania. Our colleagues in Greece—Joanna Economidou, a pediatrician and geneticist, and Stefanos Hadziyannis, a prominent figure in the hepatitis field in Europe and internationally—took part in the fieldwork and the analysis and interpretation of the data. Jean Drew, a technician in the laboratory, became interested in the gender studies and did much of the work on the analysis. Ed Lustbader developed original and imaginative statistical methods for handling what proved to be a very complex body of data.

We sampled most of the population of the community and obtained data on 326 wives and 248 husbands for a total of 390 families. We evaluated the two polar host-immune responses to the virus. An infected person either (1) becomes a carrier, remains infected for many years, and is at increased risk for the long-term effects of infection, chronic liver disease and primary cancer of the liver, or (2) develops anti-HBs, which usually confers lifelong protection against reinfection and disease. Individuals' responses at the moment of infection have a big effect on their fate: illness or health. As I have already pointed out, the males are more likely to become carriers, and the females to form anti-HBs.[14]

---

[14] It had been suggested that this might be due to the fact that during the course of their daily activities, males would be more likely to become infected and therefore more likely to become carriers. There were a variety of reasons to think that this wasn't so. Tom London's study of patients on renal dialysis provided convincing evidence. In the period before control measures were instituted, HBV infection was extremely common in renal dialysis patients because of their exposure to blood transfusions and the spread of HBV through the dialysis machines. He studied dialysis patients over several years in Philadelphia. Males and female dialysis patients were at equal risk of infection, but when infected, the males were more likely to become carriers and the females to develop anti-HBs. The differences weren't absolute, but

The sera obtained from the parents was tested to determine whether they were carriers, HBsAg(+), or had had anti-HBs. Jana and the others also collected information on the number and gender of the offspring of the tested families. The results were then arranged by the categories of families. Families were classified as (1) "carrier" families, if either parent was a carrier; (2) "antibody" families, if either parent had anti-HBs; or (3) uninfected families, if there was no evidence of HBV infection. The sex ratios were then calculated. The carrier families had a significantly higher sex ratio—more boys than girls—than the antibody families. The uninfected families were intermediate. Further, the increased sex ratio was a consequence of a decreased number of female births to the carrier mothers.

This was quite a remarkable finding. There are very few factors that disturb the sex ratio in humans; it is one of the most stable of the biological features of the species and, because of the potential effect on population size, probably affects the evolutionary history of humans. Because of the important biological implications, we tested other populations. Between 1973, when the Greek field study was accomplished, and the mid-1980s we did similar studies in Papua New Guinea, East Greenland, and Luzon, the Philippines, locations where HBV carriers were common. (We were able to use specimens collected for other purposes for these studies.) The results, in general, supported the original observations in Greece. At least one other published paper from another laboratory appeared to confirm our findings as well.

How could this be explained? Could this mean that HBV actually had an effect on the gender of its host's offspring? We formulated a variety of hypotheses. One was that there was a relation of some kind between the HBV genome and its products, on the one hand, and specific sex-determining regions on the Y chromosome (found only in men), on the other. For example, HBV might bind to this region on the Y chromosome in males but would bind less to the sex chromosomes on females, who lack the Y chromosome. This might prevent the replication of the virus in the developing male fetus, but not in a female fetus. Replication of the virus in the female fetus

there was nevertheless a high probability of differential response. At the dialysis units, the activities of men and women would be about the same.

would increase the probability of loss of the pregnancy. Therefore, in the carrier families, there would be fewer females born (as we had observed), and the sex ratio would be higher.

We also suggested a combination of behavioral characteristics and direct biological effects to explain the sex ratio observations. In many societies parents prefer sons to daughters. Consider how this preference might work itself out in the carrier families, as compared to the antibody families. In carrier families, if our data were correct, there would be a greater likelihood of having a male child. The carrier family parents might continue to have children until they had the desired number of boys—say, two. In the antibody families, there would be a higher probability of having a female child. The parents might continue to try to have children until they had achieved the desired number of boys. This would result in a larger family size and a larger proportion of females than in the carrier families.

There are possible political and social consequences of our observations on sex ratio, if they are correct and verified by other studies. The government of the People's Republic of China has for many years conducted vigorous campaigns to limit population growth. But, apparently, there is still a preference for males in Chinese culture. Professor Ansley J. Coale of Princeton University, one of the leading demographers in the United States, published a paper concerning the high sex ratios that have been observed in China. He proposed that, because there is no other biological explanation, the apparent deficit in female births in China could be a consequence of female infanticide. As might be expected, his findings and conjectures had a big play in the media. I pointed out to him that there might be a biological explanation. China, and particularly South China, has some of the highest frequencies of HBV carriers in the world. If our observations on the relation between carriers and the gender of offspring in Greece and elsewhere were also valid in China, then this might provide a biological explanation for the apparent loss of female children. Professor Coale sent one of his students to reanalyze our data, and she arrived at what appeared to be the same conclusions that we had. There has not been, as far as I know, a study of HBV and sex ratio in China, but this would clearly be useful to do, particularly since the vaccination program is moving forward in China. If the vaccination program is as effective as the early results indicate (see below for more about this), then there would be a decrease in the number of carriers within a generation. Would this decrease the sex ratio and have an effect on the desire of Chinese couples to have small families, with a preference for male offspring?

Vaccination Program: The First Successful Cancer Vaccine

The notion of a cancer vaccine is often discussed in the popular medical press. This usually means an antigen, or a substance that can produce one, that can be given to a patient with cancer to bring about a cure. At present there are no widely used and effective therapeutic cancer vaccines. In general, vaccines are essentially always used for prevention. They are given to individuals who are at risk of exposure to an infectious agent, and their risk is significantly reduced. The vaccine against HBV appears to be effective in preventing infection, and since HBV is the etiologic agent for about 85 percent of cases of hepatocellular carcinoma, it should be effective as a cancer vaccine—that is, a vaccine that prevents this common and deadly cancer. The available evidence, still preliminary, indicates that it is.

There are national HBV vaccination programs in about ninety countries. These include many of the countries in east Asia that have the highest incidence of HBV infection and HBV carriers in the world. As a consequence, about 60 percent of the population living in the high-incidence areas of the world are covered by the vaccination programs. Some of these programs have been in place for more than ten years, and it is possible to review their efficacy to see just how successful they have been. I will briefly review a sample of the reports[15] presented at the Triennial International Symposium on

[15] Some of these data are taken from a paper entitled "Cancer Prevention with a Vaccine: Hepatitis B and Liver Cancer" that I presented at the meeting of the American Association for the Advancement of Science held in Philadelphia 12–17 February 1998.

Viral Hepatitis and Liver Disease, which was held in Rome in 1996, a time when many of the vaccination programs were in place.

The public health authorities on the island of Taiwan recognized the importance of the vaccination program as soon as the vaccine became available. HBV had long been acknowledged as a major problem in Taiwan. The prevalence of HBV infection was very high: probably three-quarters of all the people on the island would become infected during the course of their lifetime. About 15 percent of the population were carriers, and in young males the prevalence was even higher. In the 1970s the morbidity and mortality reports showed that primary cancer of the liver was, in the middle age groups, the second most frequent cause of death in males—not the second-ranking cause of cancer deaths alone but the second for *all* deaths.[16]

In the early 1980s a hepatitis B control program was developed as a government-sponsored initiative.[17] Vaccine supplies were lim-

[16] I visited Taiwan in September 1978, the summer after my trip to the People's Republic of China. The health authorities had already begun the testing of blood donors—Taiwan was among the first countries to do so—and were making plans for a vaccination program. During my visit to the blood bank in Taipei I asked my hosts what they planned to do with the donor units that tested positive for HBV. They replied that the positive units were retained briefly and then discarded. I suggested that they acquire Deepfreezes and save the positive donor blood for future use in the manufacture of vaccine. When I returned to Taiwan in June of 1986, Dr. Yen Chu Tsai of the Taipei Blood Donation Center came to a seminar I was attending and asked whether I could revisit the blood bank. As we motored through the crowded summer-hot streets of the city, she told me that they now had a new center, and that other centers had been built elsewhere on Taiwan. They had followed my suggestion that they save the positive units of blood, and when the pharmaceutical companies required HBsAg for the manufacture of the blood-derived vaccine, they were able to sell the donor units and use the proceeds to build the new buildings. When we arrived at the center, I was further surprised to see my picture hanging on the wall! I spend a great deal of my time giving advice, but it still surprises me when people actually act on it. This was one of those exceptions.

[17] A review of the program is given in a paper by Ding-Shinn Chen and colleagues. (D.-S. Chen, H.-M. Hsu, C. L. Bennett, T. S. Pajeau, B. S. Blumberg, P.-Y. Chang, K. Nishioka, A. Huang, and J.-L. Sung, "A Program for Eradication of Hepatitis B from Taiwan by a 10 Year, Four-dose Vaccination Program," *Cancer Causes and Control* 7 (1996): 305–11.

ited, and it was necessary to establish a schedule of priorities for different population groups. The highest priority was given to the newborn infants of mothers who were carriers of HBV. These newborns, particularly if the virus had been actively reproducing itself—replicating—in their pregnant mother-to-be, before and around the time of birth, have a very high probability of becoming infected and remaining carriers. Palmer Beasley and his colleagues in Taiwan had reported that 86–96 percent of the newborns of carrier mothers who were replicating HBV became carriers. An infant vaccination program began on 1 July 1984. Pregnant women were tested for HBsAg; those who were positive were also tested for HBeAg to determine whether they were replicating virus. All the offspring of carrier mothers were given vaccine (which required four injections over the course of a year); if the mother was positive for HBeAg, the infants were also given immune gamma globulin.[18] In 1986, as more vaccine became available, all newborn children, irrespective of the mother's carrier state, were included. In 1987, all children under the age of five who were not among the first group vaccinated were included, and, in the same year, susceptible medical personnel as well. The following year household members of carriers were vaccinated, and in succeeding years older age groups, not previously included, were offered vaccination.

In 1989, the first part of the program had been in progress about five years, and the latter parts for a shorter period. A study of outcome was initiated. It included 255,854 of the total of 331,428 births that had been reported between July 1984 and June 1988. The prevalence of carriers in the one- to two-year age group dropped from 10.7 percent in 1984 (before the program) to 1.5 percent in 1989 (after the program). The results in selected groups were even more impressive. The prevalence in the children at highest risk, those whose mothers were actively replicating HBV, dropped from 90 percent to 15 percent. In the infants at lowest risk (whose mothers were not carriers) the unvaccinated children had a prevalence of 18 percent,

[18] Hyperimmune gamma globulin is a fraction of serum protein taken from individuals who have high titers of anti-HBs. It provides an immediate dose of antibody, anticipating the development of the antibody by the host after vaccination.

while those who were vaccinated had a prevalence of 0.2 percent, a dramatic change.

There were additional reports from other locations either presented at the Rome meeting or published elsewhere. One of the highest frequencies of HBV carriers in the United States is among Native Americans (Indians, Inuits [Eskimos], and Aleuts) resident in Alaska. Between 1981 and 1983 the U.S. Public Health Service—which, through the Indian Health Service, provides medical care for Native Americans—conducted a program to vaccinate the population. Acute hepatitis B dropped from 215 cases per 100,000[19] population before the program to 7–14 cases in 1993. In 1995 no cases were reported. This is a remarkably rapid control for a common infectious disease. Extensive programs are in place in the People's Republic of China—where 100 million carriers reside—Korea, The Gambia,[20] and elsewhere, and again the prevalence and incidence of carriers has decreased dramatically. To my knowledge, there have been no reports of systematic detrimental side effects that have stopped vaccination programs.

Italy has one of the largest numbers of HBV carriers in Europe and has been the scene of important research and application. It was one of the first European countries to have compulsory vaccination for HBV, and the results have been very encouraging. For example, a vaccination program was started in 1983 in Afragola, a community in southern Italy, near Naples, known to have a high incidence of liver disease. There were major decreases in HBV prevalence in the vaccinated population; the prevalence of HBsAg in males aged five to ten dropped from 11.9 percent in 1978 to 1.6 percent in 1989 after the vaccination program had been in place for about five years.

---

[19] Reporting cases per 100,000 is a common practice in public health; it allows comparisons of different populations. Actually, there are fewer than 100,000 Native Americans in Alaska (86,000, according to the 1990 census).

[20] The Gambia, a small West African country surrounded on three sides by Senegal, is one of several locations in Africa with a national HBV vaccination program. It is also the site of a research center of the British Medical Research Council, one of the remaining reminders of the extensive research network that existed in the colonial British Empire and Commonwealth. It is the site of a major long-term study of the effects of HBV vaccination on the incidence of HCC.

There were similar decreases in other age groups. There was an additional unexpected and curious finding in this study that has also been seen in some of the other vaccination programs. In addition to the dramatic change in carrier prevalence in the vaccinated population, there was a drop (from 13.4 percent in 1978 to 7.3 percent in 1989) in the prevalence of HBsAg and anti-HBc (another indicator of viral infection) in the *unvaccinated* population. This implies that the reduction of the carrier prevalence in the vaccinated group had an indirect effect on unvaccinated carriers and susceptibles, and that there is a decrease not only in prevalence but in incidence as well. It has been generally assumed that, once infected, most carriers will remain carriers for an indefinite period. (Actually, every year a small percentage of carriers lose their carrier status, but this is far less than the decrease observed in the Afragola study.) Does this mean that to remain a carrier, an individual has to be frequently exposed to other carriers, and that the vaccination program significantly reduced this risk? If so, how is information transmitted from the virus in one carrier to the virus in another carrier? What would be the selective advantage to the virus in decreasing titers when there are fewer carriers in the general vicinity? The answer to these fascinating evolutionary questions awaits the collection of more data.

There are other examples in the People's Republic of China, Korea, The Gambia, and elsewhere that demonstrate the considerable success of the vaccination programs. These programs have raised the possibility of the eradication of HBV, particularly if the vaccination programs can be extended to countries in Africa, south Asia, Central and South America, and elsewhere, not yet participating in vaccination programs, and if treatment for carriers becomes available. This has already been considered at the International Conference on Prospects for Eradication of HBV, held in Geneva in 1989, of which I was a co-organizer, and is likely to be raised again in the future.

The initial price of HBV vaccine was very high. As a consequence of increased international competition and other factors, the price has decreased considerably, but it is still too costly for the public health programs in many countries, particularly in sub-Saharan Africa, where the prevalence of HBV is high. Fortunately, the philanthropic foundation founded by William Gates of Microsoft and his wife is dedicating a significant portion of its very large resources to vaccination programs that include HBV. This should have a wholesome effect on the worldwide control program.

Decrease in Primary Cancer of the Liver

Even more exciting are the studies showing that the incidence of hepatocellular carcinoma is also decreasing, after only a decade of vaccination. Because of the early introduction of the vaccination program on Taiwan, some of the earliest—and most comprehensive—results have come from there. When I visited Taiwan late in 1994, I spoke with Dr. Mei-Hwei Chang, a pediatrician at the College of Public Health at the National Taiwan University. She and her colleagues were completing a survey of the effects of the HBV vaccination program on the incidence and mortality from primary cancer of the liver.

The 26 June 1997 issue of the *New England Journal of Medicine*[21] contained the report of Dr. Chang and her colleagues,[22] a concise, clear, and well-analyzed scientific paper. Taiwan has a population of 21 million and a regulated medical system in which health care is provided for all. Each citizen has a national registration number,[23] which makes possible the linking of data maintained in different databases. Chang and her coworkers obtained data from the national cancer registry, which lists all the cases of cancer in the country (and which is believed to be accurate), and from the national

---

[21] The *New England Journal of Medicine* is one of the most prestigious journals of clinical research. The acceptance of a paper by this journal imparts a cachet of importance and ensures a wide circulation.

[22] M.-H. Chang, C.-J. Chen, M.-S. Lai, H.-M. Hsu, T.-C. Wu, M.-S. Kong, D.-C. Liang, W.-Y. Shau, and D.-S. Chen, "Universal Hepatitis B Vaccination in Taiwan and the Incidence of Hepatocellular Carcinoma in Children," *New England Journal of Medicine* 336 (1997): 1855–59.

[23] This study was possible because of the existence of national IDs. At present, a national number of this sort is not legal in the United States, although the Social Security number has, to some extent, the same function. Personal and civil rights considerations have precluded the issuance of such identifiers, even for medical purposes.

death register, which gives causes of death and, again, is considered
to be accurate. They checked these against the records from the hospitals themselves to ensure accuracy.

In Taiwan, the incidence of HBV-caused cancer of the liver peaks
in the fifty- to sixty-year age group. But the disease is common, and
the incidence in young children, although much less than in adults,
is significant. The investigators decided to use the incidence of hepatocellular carcinoma between ages six and fourteen. (Disease oc-
curring in children under six might be due to another form of liver
cancer, hepatoblastoma, that is not associated with HBV.) The aver-
age annual incidence of hepatocellular carcinoma dropped from 0.7
per 100,000 population between 1981 and 1986 (before the vaccination program had started, or before it could have had an impact), to
0.57 per 100,000 between 1986 and 1990 (soon after the program had
started), and to 0.36 between 1990 and 1994. This is a statistically
significant drop. A similar and parallel drop in mortality from hepatocellular carcinoma was reflected in the death register. From 1974
to 1984 HCC was diagnosed in eighty-four children between the
ages of six and nine. In the period 1984 to 1986, the number dropped
to one. The results richly confirmed the hypothesis that HBV vaccination could prevent HCC, even when the program had been in
place for only a relatively short time.

Although the data were presented in a restrained and scholarly
style, the results are, to my mind, sensational. One of the most common cancers in the world appears to be under control. Of course,
subsequent data may change this conclusion—in science the unexpected is always looming behind the next experiment—but, on the
face of it, this appears to herald one of the most important methods
for the control of cancer. Dr. Mark Kane, who has directed hepatitis
activities at the World Health Organization, said that the vaccine
prevention of HCC is now considered to be one of the two most
important cancer control programs, exceeded only by the worldwide smoking intervention projects. According to the Centers for
Disease Control in Atlanta, HBV vaccine is the world's first anticancer vaccine;[24] we can hope that there will be others.

---

[24] Posted on the CDC website (http://www.cdc.gov) on 30 April 1998.

Back to Polymorphisms and Inherited Susceptibility to Disease

As RECOUNTED earlier in the book, the discovery of HBV emerged from our earlier research on polymorphisms, human diversity, and inherited susceptibility and resistance to disease. When we discovered HBV in 1967, we concentrated on virology, epidemiology, and clinical consequences, but the original concept of inherited susceptibility was neither ruled out nor forgotten. In this chapter, I will discuss the developments—some in our laboratory but mainly in others—that brought us back to the genetics.

Our original interest in polymorphisms began in 1956 when we started studying serum protein and other variants in several different populations, as described in chapter 3. In 1960, a few years before the discovery of HBV, I convened a conference at the National Institutes of Health on polymorphisms, susceptibility to disease, and geographic variations in disease distribution[1] and the following year published a paper[2] on the same theme. At the time of the conference there was a small band of population geneticists, anthropologists, and biologists who were working in the field. Most of them knew each other and had a certain sense of bonding as a conse-

---

[1] B. S. Blumberg, ed., *Proceedings of the Conference on Genetic Polymorphisms and Geographic Variation in Disease* (New York: Grune & Stratton, 1961).

[2] B. S. Blumberg, "Inherited Susceptibility to Disease: Its Relation to Environment," *Archives of Environmental Health* 3 (1961): 612–36.

quence of their relative intellectual isolation. In that bygone time scientists studied the polymorphisms using phenotypes, the protein product of the gene, to infer the presence of the gene itself. It was a slow and cumbersome endeavor. Since the genetic revolution it has become possible to study the polymorphisms at the DNA level by the more rapid methods of molecular biology. This has given birth to a whole new science—genomics—fathered and mothered by the Human Genome Project. There is also a developing field of proteomics, the study of the protein variants produced by the DNA variants. Strangely, the field is returning to where we left off with it! But let's go back to retracing the story of the genetic studies and how they relate to susceptibility and resistance to chronic infection with HBV.

In chapter 6, I described the family studies with which, in the 1960s, we tested the hypothesis that Australia antigen was a serum protein polymorphism segregating at a locus we termed *Au*. We continued to test the genetic hypothesis even after we discovered the virus, but altered it to say that we were attempting to identify the genes that conferred increased susceptibility or resistance to persistent infection with the virus. The trait was difficult to study: if a person had inherited the susceptibility genotype but was not exposed to HBV, the genotype could not be revealed and the expected segregation pattern would be only partially fulfilled. Also, the ability to become a carrier was age- and gender-dependent and related to other factors in the environment. In the 1980s Ed Lustbader took the project up again and did a sophisticated analysis of Chinese families in which he took account of some of these variables. As predicted, the data were consistent with a genetic susceptibility to persistent infection. Ed's untimely death left the project uncompleted.

Further progress on the genetics of HBV had to wait until the molecular biology and virology caught up with the biology. This has now happened. Molecular biology has enormously increased the possibilities of discovering polymorphisms because the methods can be used to identify the very common genetic variations in the base pair sequences. Polymorphisms have become important in the

Human Genome Project because they are used to map the location of major genes, including those that cause inherited disease, and to construct the gene maps that will be among the main products of the Project. Automated methods now permit the rapid identification of variation and polymorphisms. In the past, the discovery of a polymorphism and its relation to diseases could be a multiyear project. Now, many polymorphisms can be identified in the course of a few days.

Progress on the genetics of HBV continued along the convoluted path that you have by now become accustomed to. Adrian Hill was appointed the Huxley Royal Society Research Fellow at Balliol College while I was the Master (1989–94). I was pleased with his appointment because he was working on polymorphisms and disease susceptibility to malaria and other infectious diseases, a subject close to my own interests. Adrian and I organized a seminar on population biology that convened in the dining room of my lodgings at the college. It was an excellent forum that brought together outstanding scientists in the field at Oxford who were ordinarily spread over many departments and different sites. It also provided an opportunity for me to follow the research Adrian was doing at the British Medical Research Council laboratory in Banjul, The Gambia, West Africa. I will describe a small part of what they and others in the field have accomplished.

The major histocompatibility complex (MHC) consists of a series of gene loci situated near each other on human chromosome 6. The class II MHC genes produce proteins that present antigens, processed from foreign materials that enter the body, to the host immune cells. These immune cells, T cells and B cells, can then produce an immune response to the foreign material and help to reject it. The multiple genes in this group are highly polymorphic—that is, there are many different alleles at each of the loci. So the responses mediated by these loci are complex and highly individualized. They have been important in transplantation surgery: close matches of some of the MHC proteins between the organ donor and the patient recipient are required to decrease the probability that a transplant will be rejected. The MHC proteins have a similar role in dealing with the foreign proteins introduced to a putative host by viruses and other microorganisms.

Adrian, his colleague Mark Thurz from St. Mary's Hospital in London, and their Gambian and other coworkers examined the relation between MHC polymorphisms and the clinical response to infection with malaria caused by *Plasmodium falciparum*. *P. falciparum* is the most deadly of the malaria parasites and a very common killer of children in West Africa. They identified individuals in the study population who had become infected with the malaria parasite; patients who developed cerebral malaria—a major cause of the childhood deaths from *P. falciparum*—were distinguished from those who had not, and the MHC alleles were determined in each of the patient groups. The investigators found a significant association with one of the alleles (or *haplotypes*, since they reflect alleles at several of the linked loci) in MHC class II. Infected persons, particularly children, who have inherited the allele DRB1*1302 (as might be expected, the nomenclature of these alleles is complex) are significantly *less* likely to develop the cerebral from of malaria than those with other alleles at this locus. This is an important finding; anything that can be learned about the pathogenesis of cerebral malaria and its prevention could help to alleviate the misery caused by this scourge of young children. In this instance, the polymorphism was related not to susceptibility to the initial infection with the malaria organism but to the *response* of the human host after the infection. Adrian and the others are using this information in a program to develop a vaccine based on the specific malaria antigens that are presented by the MHC proteins.

I think that it was, at least in part, because of our discussions of HBV that Adrian and Mark looked at the relation of the MHC polymorphism to the response to infection with HBV. There was already a great deal of information on HBV at the MRC laboratory in Banjul, since it is the site of a major epidemiology program on HBV vaccination. They found that DRB1*1302, the same MHC class II allele that was associated with protection against cerebral malaria, conferred relative protection against developing the carrier state for HBV! (There was also an association with DRB1*1301.) In addition, they found that individuals who developed cerebral malaria had a higher likelihood of also being carriers of HBV. So there was a connection between these two organisms that might have importance in malaria and HBV control, and also in the development of medications for one, the other, or both.

This isn't the end of the story but rather the beginning. Within the past few years other polymorphisms have been identified that are related to the response to HBV. Before getting too far into this discussion, I should caution you that this field is still young, and many of the studies are based on small samples and often have not been validated. Since the distribution of polymorphic alleles varies greatly from one population to another—that was the theme of many of our field studies in the 1950s and 1960s—associations may be found in some populations and not in others. While an association between an allele and a disease might occur in one population, it might not occur in another because environmental factors that interact with the gene and the host may exist in the first and be absent or diminished in the second. Also, the gene pools in individuals and populations differ, and that too can affect the associations.

The polymorphism connections that have been identified have been quite unexpected; it would have been difficult before the event to predict which polymorphisms might be related to HBV, but after they have been identified, a hypothesis to explain the relation can always be formulated and experiments devised to test it. I will briefly describe some of the other HBV-related susceptibility and resistance genes to illustrate the unpredictable and complex associations that have been found.

The VDR locus on Chromosome 12 controls the production of the vitamin D receptor protein. One of VDR's functions is to bind a metabolite of vitamin D that regulates calcium metabolism. There are several polymorphic sites on the VDR gene, one of which is designated *T*; two alleles segregate at this locus, *T* and *t*. Persons who are homozygous for the *t* allele, *tt*, have a decreased probability of becoming carriers if infected with HBV. This same locus is related to the response to infection with *Mycobacterium leprae*, the causative bacteria of Hansen's disease (leprosy); the *tt* homozygote is less likely to develop lepromatous leprosy and more likely to develop tuberculoid leprosy[3] than persons who have inherited the alternative alleles. The *tt* homozygotes have, in general, lower bone mineral density and are more prone to develop osteoporosis. They are also at lower risk for cancer of the prostate.

The mannose-binding protein (MBP) is a serum protein in mammals that binds the sugar mannose present in glycoproteins[4] on the surface of certain bacteria and other disease-causing agents. This leads to the destruction of the microorganism and its take-up by opsonizing (engulfing) cells in the host. The gene controlling this protein is located on chromosome 10, and it has several polymorphic sites. An allele at this locus is associated with an increased susceptibility to becoming a carrier of HBV. There are also alleles that are associated with a rapid onset of the symptoms of AIDS in persons infected with HIV, the causative virus for the disease. Another allele at the MBP locus is associated with susceptibility to the autoimmune disease systemic lupus erythematosus.

Tumor necrosis factor (TNF) is a cytokine (one of a class of proteins or glycoproteins involved in the regulation of cellular proliferation and function) that has many roles, including control of inflammation and stimulation of the proliferation and destruction of cancer cells. It also increases cachexia (severe wasting and weight loss) in cancer patients, a strange and not fully understood phenomenon. There are several polymorphic sites on the TNF gene. They are related to susceptibility to HBV chronicity, cerebral malaria, lepromatous leprosy, and a form of the tropical disease caused by the protozoan *Leishmania braziliensis*. There are several other polymorphic loci—about five—that influence susceptibility to chronic infection with HBV, but the examples given provide a notion of the richness of the system.

What of the gene we postulated years ago, Au^1, which in homozygous form increased the individual's risk of becoming a carrier? Is

---

[3] Leprosy can occur in at least two different clinical forms. Lepromatous leprosy is usually more systemic and difficult to treat. Tuberculoid leprosy is usually manifested more on the skin, is less aggressive, and is easier to treat.

[4] Glycoproteins are proteins that are combined with sugars.

it actually one of the polymorphisms that have been identified and described above? Adrian Hill and his colleagues are trying to identify the postulated Au^1 gene through studies in families with multiple carriers of HBV.[5]

Meanwhile, from the data we have on the susceptibility genes for HBV, some interesting inferences and conjectures can be made that have broad implications in medicine. There are a few leitmotifs threading through the big orchestration I am attempting to put together. It is useful to distinguish between (1) the major genes that determine inherited diseases (*monogenetic* diseases), and (2) polymorphic susceptibility and resistance genes. The major genes, with some exceptions, tend to be rare—one in a few hundred or a few thousand people—and the diseases they cause constitute a relatively small part of the human disease load. They are "penetrant"— that is, if the gene is present (in single dose if it is a dominant gene or in double dose if it is a recessive gene), then there is a high likelihood that the disease will be manifest in the person who has inherited the genes. The major genes are *deterministic* in the sense that if the gene is present, there is a high probability that the disease will develop.

Polymorphic alleles, on the other hand, are common in the population; the allele at a polymorphic locus at lowest frequency will be present in 2–3 percent, or more, of the population. Polymorphisms are associated with the common illnesses—heart disease, cancer, infectious diseases, and the like—that are the major causes of human morbidity and mortality. Susceptibility genes are less penetrant; often an environmental factor must be present for the effect of the gene to be realized, and the environmental effects may be far more important than the inherited factors. For example, the susceptibility genes for HBV chronicity will not have an observable effect unless

---

[5] I wrote to my colleague Professor Alberto Vierruci of the University of Florence to ask whether we could collaborate on this study. As always, he was enthusiastic about the project. He told me, however, that while it had been possible to identify families with multiple carriers twenty years ago when we were at the beginning of our research, it was now difficult to do so because the vaccination program had been so effective. This was very good news, despite the fact that it would slow down the project.

the bearer of the genes is also infected with HBV. Hence the polymorphic susceptibility genes are not deterministic. Nearly all genes
are subject to environmental effects, but the susceptibility genes
more so than the major genes. Major genes often act on their own;
susceptibility genes act in concert with environmental agents and
with other genes.

One of the societal concerns with the Human Genome Project has
been the presumed deterministic character of genes. If all the genes
are known, it is argued, then life outcomes will be totally predictable
and even controllable. Pessimistic science fiction scenarios picture a
future world in which people with optimal genomes will be favored, and those with less desirable configurations will have a diminished role in society. The possibility that humans might be
cloned and the possibility that genomes could be designed with
traits that are deemed by some to be desirable have raised great debates at the national and international level.

It is useful to review the lessons gained from the growing knowledge of susceptibility genes. They are less deterministic, and far
more complex, than the genes of monogenetic diseases. They act in
concert, they interact with the environment, and there is scope for
intervention. The effects of the susceptibility genes are influenced
by the total genetic pool of the individual and of the population of
which he or she is a part. In addition, the same susceptibility gene
may have both advantageous and disadvantageous effects. For example the *tt* homozygote at the VDR gene may be advantageous in
that it protects against chronicity of HBV and the development of
cerebral malaria, but disadvantageous in that it increases the probability of osteoporosis. There are many such examples in the genome.
Susceptibility genes cannot be classified simply as "good" or "bad":
they may be good under some circumstances and bad under others.
Again, it reminds us that evolution leads not to perfection but to
"getting by"; it requires diversity in the gene pool. If a genome is
perfect for the present environment, then it may be less so for an
environment that may develop in the future. Greater diversity
allows a population to be prepared for a very wide variety of future
environments, many of which cannot be predicted on the basis of
the past.

This topic is reminiscent of the age-old philosophical debate concerning determinism and free will. While many individual genetic processes may be deterministic, their combinations involve so many possibilities and so many opportunities for human-willed intervention that the overall effect is the equivalent of free will.[6] It is these considerations that make the study of chaos and complexity theory such an interesting and rapidly developing field of academic and applied research.

The target date for the conclusion of the Human Genome Project is about 2003; a "first draft" was presented in 2000. Upon its completion, all the human genes will have been identified, and the sequence of the entire genome established. The functions of most of the genes will still not be known, particularly since genes have multiple functions; the complex interactions, of which the illustrations I have given are but a minuscule fraction, will also be unknown. The new disciplines—genomics and proteomics—are emerging. They are information-based systems that could reveal the genetic characteristics of an individual and of populations, and how these relate to the environment and to health and disease. Knowledge of the specific susceptibility alleles carried by an individual could lead

---

[6] The 1997 sci-fi movie *Gattaca* has an interesting take on the notion of genes and fate. It posits a future world where individuals are selected at birth to have an ideal genome, either by choice of gametes or by alteration of their gene pool. The hero, Vincent Freeman, who is born without undergoing this process, is judged inferior and not allowed to become an astronaut and venture to Titan, the Saturnian moon, to fulfill his lifelong ambition. However, he encounters Jerome, a genetically perfected young man who, because of an accidental injury, is leading an indolent life. Vincent fakes Jerome's genes by substituting Jerome's blood and other tissues for genetic testing when he has to enter the precincts of Gattaca Corporation, the company organizing the space flights. It all gets a little complicated when there is a murder. Vincent's efforts are nearly thwarted, and Uma Thurman—who enjoys the unusual distinction of having the letters of her first name appear in the same order in her last—playing Irene Cassini, the Arctic-cold heroine of the drama, gets embroiled in the mix. Well, Vincent prevails, goes to Titan, and demonstrates that genes aren't everything, that biology isn't destiny, that the genetical planners don't know it all— because the combination of genes, environment, and the exercise of the will is what really counts. The tag line for the film is "There is no gene for the human spirit," a wholesome thought.

to the design of protective interventions, or could help in the prediction of disease and its avoidance. There is the rosy promise of a longer life unimpeded by serious illness.

The potential problems of this technology are already raising concerns. How much do we want to know about our biology, particularly if practical intervention is not possible? Will a person identified as susceptible to a specific disease, even when the susceptibility is expressed in terms of probabilities, be denied employment or health and life insurance, or even become socially ostracized? The developing science generates intense spikes of both hope and fear. It will be exciting to see what emerges from all this ferment within the next few decades.

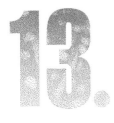

HBV and Its Connections: Current Research and the Future

SCIENCE is a forward-looking endeavor. Scientists build on the past—as we built on the firm groundwork of research that preceded ours—but their thoughts are on the results of the next experiment and the one beyond that. Writing this narrative caused to me to reflect on the rich events, both personal and scientific, that were part of the discovery quest, and I hope that I have conveyed some of the excitement to you. I completed this account in the millennium (if you agree that 2000 is the actual millennium year), during which I celebrated my seventy-fifth birthday along with many of my friends born in 1925. It was an appropriate time for this summing up.

In this final chapter, I will review some of the recent work undertaken by many scientists worldwide who have advanced knowledge about HBV far beyond our meager beginnings. These pages are intended to bring the story, briefly, up to the present, and to make some guesses about the future. I won't attempt to describe everything that is happening in the hepatitis field, which has enlarged greatly as more scientists have worked in it, but will deal with some subjects of special and curious interest.

HCV and Other Hepatitis Viruses

I have occasionally referred to hepatitis C virus (HCV) and other hepatitis viruses. They were discovered after HBV, but their story is intermixed with the HBV saga because they have an affinity for the liver and cause similar symptoms and pathology. As HBV has begun to come under control through prevention and, to some extent, treatment, there has been an increased focus on other hepatitis viruses.

After the identification of HBV there was an intense search for the virus spread by the fecal-oral route—that is, the ingestion of infected human waste—whose existence had been recognized by Saul Krugman and many other investigators well before the discovery of HBV. Within a few years of the discovery of HBV, hepatitis A virus was found in the stools of victims, excellent methods of detection were devised, and, in time, an effective vaccine was invented. The military and travelers to locations where sanitation is poor, and the likelihood of fecal contamination of food and water is high, now use the vaccine widely. In some jurisdictions many others use it as well. In recent years there have been concerns, in the United States and elsewhere, about the integrity of the water supply and food cleanliness. The availability of a vaccine for a common contaminant of human waste is a real comfort, although prevention by ensuring the security of the water and food supply, is, of course, the best strategy. HAV is a common cause of acute hepatitis but is only rarely chronic. The carrier state is rare, and HAV is not associated with the pathogenesis of hepatocellular carcinoma. It is an RNA virus in a family quite distinct from the Hepadna viruses, which include HBV and the other animal viruses that are similar to HBV.

After HAV and HBV had been identified, it became clear that there were other blood-borne and fecal-oral hepatitis viruses. The next discovery (by Dr. Mario Rizzetto in Turin in 1977) was hepatitis D virus (HDV). It is the smallest known human viral pathogen—it has only seventeen hundred base pairs—and it infects only people who are also infected with HBV. HDV uses the handy device of coating itself in a protein that is very similar to the HBsAg that coats HBV. To the outside world, it masquerades as an HBV virus, but deep down it has its own antigens, nucleic acid, and unique methods of replication and pathogenesis. It can cause severe disease, including fulminant hepatitis, a particularly virulent form of the disease that can kill within days or weeks.

HDV has an interesting distribution. It is very common in HBV-positive intravenous drug users in the United States, in many parts of Europe, and elsewhere. It is difficult to arrive at a convincing explanation for this, but it raises the possibility that IV drug users form an unusual "blood brotherhood" because of frequent sharing of needles and the rapid transport of people from one place to another in the jet age. HDV is also quite common in HBV carriers in several countries in Africa and in the Amazon region of Brazil. Fortunately the HBV vaccine protects against infection with HDV.

It soon became apparent there were other viruses in addition to A, B, and D. There were still blood-borne cases of hepatitis and huge epidemics of apparently water- and food-transmitted hepatitis that could not be assigned to any of the three known viruses. There followed a dogged race to identify the unknown viruses. Daniel Bradley and his colleagues at the Centers for Disease Control in Atlanta identified the presence of a blood-borne virus different from HBV in a series of animal and laboratory experiments. In 1989, Michael Houghton, Qui-Lim Choo, and others at the Chiron Corporation—a biotech company—used the serum of convalescent patients to screen for the DNA of the virus and identified a portion of it. On the basis of this work, an effective diagnostic was developed that was quickly applied to the screening of donor blood. This greatly reduced the residue of posttransfusion hepatitis that remained after the introduction of screening for HBV had been instituted in the 1970s.

With the availability of an accurate diagnostic test, the extent of the HCV "epidemic" became apparent. Many cases of chronic hepatitis whose causes had not been known were diagnosed as HCV. HCV is now the main reason for liver transplants in the United States. An even greater shock was in store. The HCV diagnostic test made possible the detection of occult (asymptomatic) cases. It was estimated, from population surveys, that there were more than four million carriers of HCV in the United States alone! By comparison, there had been one million or more HBV carriers before the vaccination and other control measures were in place, and it is likely that the number of HBV infections will decrease in time as vaccination programs continue to be implemented. Extensive studies of the natural history of HCV indicated that initial infection was often followed by a long asymptomatic period (of years or even decades), and that a significant percentage of those infected eventually developed chronic infection and chronic liver disease. Researchers took histories to find out how infection occurred. A large percentage, probably 50 percent or more, of the study population became infected by using injectable—usually illegal—drugs. Even a small number of needle exposures in the 1960s or 1970s could have been the source of the infection that was diagnosed twenty to thirty years later.

Many of the cases (both HBV and HCV) were a consequence of the widespread experimentation with injectable drugs common in the 1960s and 1970s. What a terrible irony! A youthful period of experimentation, with no health consequences obvious at the time, came back to threaten the health and life of the adult now with spouse, children, jobs, and all the accompaniments of a settled life. I had many calls from patients and families of patients distressed by the news, often after a routine blood test, that they were infected with HCV or HBV. There are treatments available, but they are not effective in all cases. Nor is there a vaccine for HCV, although a great deal of research is currently ongoing in an effort to invent one. Of course, not all the cases are due to IV drug use. Before screening of blood donors for HCV was possible, and before the availability of disposable needles and other medical equipment, the virus could have been transmitted iatrogenically (induced by physicians) or nosocomially (in a hospital setting). And in many cases the mode of transmission is unknown. In the beginning years of the twenty-first century, HCV is one of the major infectious diseases in the United States. Worldwide, there are more carriers of HBV (about 350 million) than HCV (about 150–200 million). Taken together, the hepatitis viruses are among the most common infectious agents of humankind.

HEV, a virus that is spread by contaminated food and water, has also been identified. HEV epidemics are somewhat similar to those of HAV; before the identification of HAV, HBV, HCV, and HDV, the epidemics could not easily be distinguished from one another. HEV was found to be the cause of major epidemics, often in Asia, that would affect hundreds of individuals when drinking water and food became contaminated with untreated sewage. There were often many deaths; tragically, in these epidemics, young pregnant woman were particularly prone to a fatal outcome.

There is no vaccine against HEV, and the best preventive would be protection of water and food from contamination with human waste. Many other killing infectious diseases are also spread by contaminated food and water. A program to improve waste disposal and provide clean water would be one of the most important health measures in most developing countries. If combined with the control of disease-carrying mosquitoes and available vaccinations, these straightforward public health measures could transform the health status and economy of many countries now laboring under a crushing burden of disease.

In 1986 I spent an extended period of time in India serving as the Raman Professor at the Indian Institute of Sciences, in Bangalore, a major city in the southern province of Karnataka. In addition to other responsibilities I undertook a survey of the hepatitis problem. I believe that the major reason I was asked to do this was to provide information on the need for and production of HBV vaccine. I spoke with senior health officials, academic leaders, and the prime minister, Rajiv Gandhi.[1] It was clear from my investigation of the problem that a vaccination program was only part of what was needed. In my report to the prime minister and the health officials, submitted in the spring of 1986, I recommended, in addition to the vaccination program, the establishment of schools of public health, the development of resources for the manufacture of disposable needles and syringes, and the introduction of a massive program for the improvement of the water supply and the disposal of human waste. I often wondered whether my intercession had much of an effect.

Human Immunodeficiency Virus (HIV) and AIDS

The hepatitis viruses are, as I have detailed, major causes of disease and death. But while the discoveries of HBV and the other hepatitis viruses were in progress, another terrible disease intruded itself forcibly into the consciousness of the world. The tragic story of HIV is well known; during the last half of the twentieth century

---

[1] The prime minister had been a pilot for Indian Airlines for many years and understood technology. He was remarkably well informed about the hepatitis problem. Sadly, he was assassinated several months after our visit.

no disease attracted as much attention, concern, and public support for its control. In the early 1980s several young men in urban centers in the United States developed rapidly progressive infections for which they could not muster a sufficient immunological response. They were defenseless against a series of infectious agents against which they would ordinarily have been naturally protected. Very soon after the appearance of this disease, its viral cause was determined. It was a hitherto unknown virus, HIV, that reproduced itself through the reverse transcriptase mode—that is, the RNA produced DNA during the course of the replication cycle. Even before the virus was discovered, the modes of infection could be inferred. Its epidemiology is strikingly similar to that of HBV: it is transmitted sexually, by transfusion, by injection (for example, illicit drug use, nondisposable medical needles, reused medical equipment that is exposed to blood), and by other mechanisms in which blood can be transfused from one individual to the next. The disease spread very rapidly and soon became one of the great killers in the United States, Europe, Africa, Southeast Asia, and elsewhere. It now is a major cause of mortality worldwide.

Attempts to control the transmission followed a pattern similar to that pioneered with HBV. A reliable diagnostic was developed, and all transfusion donor blood was tested—but, unfortunately, only in countries that could afford this public health luxury. This essentially stopped the transmission by transfusion in those more fortunate countries. This did not happen in time to prevent the transmission of HIV to a very large proportion of the hemophilia population. Hemophilia patients were periodically given antihemophilia globulin (AHG), a blood product that was derived from a very large donor pool. The large size of the pool nearly guaranteed that one or more of the donors would be infected with HIV; a single blood could contaminate a whole batch of AHG that, in turn, could be administered to many patients.

The importance of using disposable needles was already known from the experience with HBV; in some regions the AIDS epidemic accelerated the demand for these products and, indirectly, contributed to the decrease in HBV and HCV infection. The knowledge that this deadly disease could be transmitted sexually had a profound social impact. Topics of sexuality that had not previously been broadly discussed became the subjects of widely disseminated public information programs directed to both adults and the young— for example, the use of contraceptive sheaths, and counseling against promiscuity and multiple partners. It was said that AIDS stopped the "sexual revolution" that had flourished in the guilt- and (relatively) venereal disease–free 1960s and 1970s.

Dentists suddenly confronted their patients wearing face shields, masks, gloves, and other devices for protection against the possibility of blood-borne transmission. All these measures helped to decrease the transmission of HBV and HCV as well as HIV. In fact, the effect on the hepatitis viruses was probably greater: HBV is more easily transmitted and is hardier than HIV. HIV can also be transmitted from infected mothers to their newborn children, although the probability of transmission is much less than for HBV. Fortunately, treatment of the mother with antiviral agents can considerably decrease the incidence of transmission.

A vaccine for AIDS has not yet been invented, but not for lack of trying. More is known about the virology of HIV, the mode of replication and transmission, and the features of its molecular soul than about any other virus that has been studied. But, ironically, this has not been sufficient to enable scientists to devise a protective vaccine. Yet the mood remains hopeful, and the large amount of energy and effort dedicated to HIV research is likely to result in success.

Many more people have died, worldwide, of HBV and HCV than of AIDS, although the annual death rates for the latter continue to rise in parts of the world. Why, then, has there been a greater fear of AIDS than of HBV? The first cases of AIDS were diagnosed before the virus had been identified, and when the patients were nearing the end of their clinical course. Hence the diagnosis was associated with rapid and nearly universal death. It wasn't until the virus was discovered that it became apparent that the disease had a long (seven to ten years or more) incubation period after infection, but even then the high mortality rate and the lack of effective therapy remained very grave aspects of the disease. HBV infection, on the other hand, was often associated in the public mind with an acute infectious disease from which patients nearly always recovered. Not until the discovery of Australia antigen—which made it possible for doctors to diagnose carriers and patients with chronic liver disease and cancer of the liver—did the deadly nature of the virus became apparent. By that time, the HBV vaccine was available, and several reasonably good therapies were in use. There was a tacit assumption that the disease was under control, although this was (and is) far from the case. However, the research on AIDS has been of indirect benefit to the scientists working on HBV and the other hepatitis viruses. It has resulted in a great increase in our knowledge of viruses in general and has focused the attention of the pharmaceutical companies on antiviral medications.

The Future

The process of our research was indirect, winding through circuitous paths, ideas, places, and involving many people, but it had a curious order, vector, and a satisfactory outcome. The search isn't over, though; basic research never is. Here is a short discussion of ideas and conjectures for the future.

Are there other virus-cancer relations that can be tackled by the interventional methods learned from the HBV-HCC relation? The answer to this must be "Yes" since other virus-cancer relations are already known or suspected—for example, the probable etiologic relation between human papilloma virus and carcinoma of the cervix of the uterus—and it is likely that many more will be found in the future. How do the HBV genes that are integrated into human cell genomes affect the transcription of other human genes? Viral diseases, including HBV, are known to have mental effects, such as depression, malaise, and loss of appetite. Can changes in human gene transcription caused by the viral genes alter the mental state and behavior of the host? If so, can this line of research help toward a better understanding of the relation of genes to behavior?

There is still a great need for an antiviral for HBV despite the availability of interferon—a drug that acts, in part, by enhancing the immune response to a virus—and of other therapies currently under test. The rapid growth in the knowledge of the molecular biology of HBV has revealed many pathways where therapeutic intervention is possible. My colleagues Professor Raymond Dwek, director of the Glycobiology Institute at Oxford University, and Timothy Block at Thomas Jefferson University Medical School in Philadelphia have, for several years, studied the effects of a synthetic sugar that inhibits the glycosylation process of HBsAg.[2] This appears to alter the structure of the surface antigen and the assembly of the virus, and to inhibit the export of the virus from the liver cells, which, in turn, could slow down the pathogenic pathway. They are now trying to determine whether this has therapeutic value. There are many other sites where medications could be helpful—for example, the inhibition of the viral DNA polymerase and reverse transcriptase that are required for the replication of the virus. My guess is that it will be very difficult to totally eliminate HBV from liver cells, because integration of the viral DNA is common. However, it may be possible to effect what we have called "treatment by delay." HBV is a patient virus; it remains in its carrier host for three, four, or even five decades without causing any perceptible trouble. A goal of "therapy" would be to delay the onset of symptoms in the carrier so that the asymptomatic period would prevail still longer, and the host could live out his or her expected life span and die of some other disease. Meanwhile, in populations protected by the vaccine, the incidence and prevalence of HBV should gradually decrease or even, conceivably, disappear.

What is the effect of the interaction of HBV with other microorganisms it finds inside the host that it invades? Does it alter the response to HIV, to malaria, to HCV, and to the many other microorganisms that share the same external and internal environment? Does this impact prevention and treatment strategies? How many of these organisms, environmental factors, hosts, and genes acting in a grand polyphonic symphony can we comprehend and analyze? Is there a limit to the complexity that humans can intellectually

---

[2] The means by which sugar molecules are attached to the surface antigen protein (HBsAg).

manage? There is still plenty to engage the thoughts and time of generations of scientists yet unborn.

Hepatitis has been a terrible affliction of humans, and it is very gratifying to all who have worked in this field to see that the problem has begun to yield to research and development. Deaths from acute fulminant hepatitis, from liver failure, and from primary cancer of the liver are terrible to suffer and to witness; "victories" against one of the perpetrators—HBV—are very welcome. Let us hope that there will be even more successes. However, I have spent a good part of my professional life studying HBV and have developed a certain level of admiration for this genetically challenged four-reading-framed organism that is only arguably living. It has managed to thrive in a certain harmony with its host, devising mechanisms for survival that we would not have imagined had we not learned of them from HBV itself. We can hope that the knowledge gained in the study of HBV will help in the control of other noxious agents.

In 1999, just before the millennium descended upon us, my scientific life took an unusual and unexpected change in direction. I was appointed director of the National Aeronautics and Space Administration (NASA) Astrobiology Institute (NAI) and, as such, became involved in one of the grandest research programs of all time. The mission of the astrobiology enterprise, of which the NAI is a part, is to study the origins, evolution, and destiny of life on Earth and in the universe—no mean task. It is part of an even larger NASA program—Origins—whose goal is, as the NASA pronouncements put it, "The Search for our Cosmic Roots by the Study of Galaxies, Stars, Planets . . . and Life." The scientists involved in this project include astronomers, molecular biologists, geologists, paleontologists, microbiologists, planetary scientists, biologists, cosmologists, physicists, chemists, and many others. NAI is charged with the study of primitive organisms—such as the archaea that live in the hot springs of Yellowstone and adjacent to the lava vents and black smokers found at the juncture of the tectonic plates in the depths of the world's oceans—that may be related to the earliest organisms on earth. It supports studies on the earliest microfossils, on the possibility of evidence of past life in meteorites that arrived from Mars millions of years ago and landed in the vast coldness of the Antarctic. The program encompasses research on the molecular biology of cells and organisms in space growing in near-zero gravity, and on the formation of pre-RNA and protein molecules in or on the infant Earth or elsewhere. A prime mission is the development of methods for the detection of life on planets and moons in our solar system—particularly Mars and Europa, the moon of Jupiter that is thought to have large quantities of water—or on planets circling other stars, light-years away from our home on Earth and even the cozy environment of the Milky Way galaxy. The facilities available are incredible. An orbiting space laboratory has been incorporated into the International Space Station; various satellites and land-based telescopes are in place or will be launched to find and study the biospheres of distant planets; there will be robotic (and, possibly, human) missions to Mars, to Europa, and to comets, to collect stardust; and many other incredible engineering and scientific tasks will be undertaken. NAI will, if we can manage it, be a basic scientific organization whose goal it will be to increase our knowledge of nature and help to answer the scientific and metaphysical questions "How did we get here?" "Are we alone?" and "What is the future of humans in space?"[3]

It is a big step from the study of one of the smallest human pathogens to the cosmic questions of space and time. While, in my mind, roaming the vastness of the universe, I will continue to heed the lessons about the grand design of nature taught by this virus hovering on the borders of life.

[3] Taken, in part, from the *Third Annual State of Origins Report* (NASA, 17 May 1999).

Appendix 1

Scientists and Staff at Fox Chase
Cancer Center Referred to in the Text

I HAVE referred to many members of Fox Chase Cancer Center who were involved in the hepatitis research. In this appendix additional information is provided on several of them.

Ann Dortort was the secretary of our research group, the Division of Clinical Research of Fox Chase Cancer Center, for most of the period described in the book. She really became the executive director in the sense that she may have been the only member of the group who had a comprehensive idea of what we were doing and where everyone was. She was a faultless secretary at a time, before the advent of word processors, when secretaries had to type and retype letters and scientific manuscripts. It is hard to believe, but I do not recall ever finding a typing error in Ann's products.

Ann had always wanted to be a secretary and became one soon after graduating from high school and attending secretarial school. After she had been in our division for several years, she obtained a bachelor's degree, attending LaSalle University in Philadelphia weekends and summers. She did a brilliant senior paper on the migration history of Philadelphia. She even talked the president of the university into awarding me an honorary degree, so Ann and I "graduated" at the same time.

Ann trained the secretaries who subsequently joined the division, Maureen Climaldi and Joyce Codispoti, who learned excellence from her; they have become leaders in their own right. She remembered everyone's birthday and made sure that they were celebrated; she was the spirit of the division.

W. Thomas London is a physician trained at Cornell University Medical School. We first met at the National Institutes of Health, where he worked in an epidemiology group allied to mine. Tom is bright; he always seems to grasp the fundamental biological principles more readily than I. Frequently, I would visit Tom after a particularly esoteric lecture to make sure I knew what the speaker was talking about. He also had an extraordinary memory and could place a particular experiment in the appropriate historical context to see where we should go next. Perhaps his greatest contribution was his scientific imagination. He would come forward with the most intriguing hypotheses and then design the appropriate studies to test them. Tom took over the direction of the research group after I left FCCC for Oxford in 1989, and he has continued with fascinating and complex projects on HBV and cancer.

Alton Sutnick is a clinician and laboratory scientists trained at the University of Pennsylvania who came to us from the Department of Medicine at Temple University. He was an excellent physician. In addition, he had an extraordinary capacity for seeing the dimensions of a problem, deciding how to resolve it, and then proceeding relentlessly until the work was finished. With Al, once the train was on the track, you could be sure that it would quickly and effectively arrive at the next station. If there were new methods to be learned, he would learn them; if new concepts were needed, he would acquire them as well. He went on to become the dean of the Medical College of Pennsylvania, a post he occupied with great distinction for many years.

Irving Millman obtained his Ph.D. degree in immunology and immunochemistry. He was the only one in our group with any formal advanced training in microbiology and virology. After a period in academic institutions, he was employed at the Merck Institute for Therapeutic Research, one of whose laboratories was located near Philadelphia. While there, he perfected an excellent vaccine for pertussis. Irving was instrumental in the development of our hepatitis B vaccine. Having had prior experience with vaccines, he was able to outline the procedures to be used once we had decided on the general approach. His contributions were recognized when, in 1993, the vaccine and radioimmunoassay patents and their inventors (Irving and me) were elected to the National Inventors Hall of Fame, an unusual honor for a medical invention. Irving was proficient in developing laboratory methods and helped direct the laboratory in the techniques of molecular biology when these became available.

Lisa Melartin Prehn, from the University of Turku in western Finland, was one of the first scientists to arrive at the Philadelphia laboratory. Graduates of Scandinavian medical schools are required to complete a significant research project and write a thesis before they are awarded the M.D. degree. They often go abroad to find the laboratory facilities in which to undertake their research, and Lisa chose to come to my laboratory to work on serum protein polymorphisms. She did an excellent thesis on a polymorphism of serum albumin that she discovered, but also did many of the laboratory and field studies in the early stages of the research on Australia antigen. Lisa was the first of a series of Finnish scientists who came to work at Fox Chase Cancer Center. She invited one or two to succeed her, and they or she would always manage to recommend excellent scientists who would come to work with us when their predecessors left. The Finnish *sisu* became a code word in the laboratory. It is difficult to translate; it means, I think, dogged determination against mighty odds to prevail. It was much used in descriptions of the Finnish character during the bitter war against the Russian invasion before and during World War II. In the laboratory, it was applied to the hard work required to complete a long series of tests, often frustrating, that required active patience to see the project through. We still have a large group of old friends and coworkers in the far north of Europe.

Barbara Werner was one of the first technicians who came to the laboratory. She was involved in the earliest discoveries, in particular in the genetics of the HBV carrier state. She isolated the serum fraction that was used when the first electron microscope images of an HBV particle were obtained, and was responsible for a large proportion of the data in the HBV and cancer studies. Barbara developed a strong sense of independence in her work, which we encouraged. This led to an interesting consequence that has been related in the text. In time, she recognized that to advance and develop a separate scientific identity, she would require a graduate degree. She went to Western Reserve University, obtained a Ph.D. in immunology, and returned to our laboratory briefly before taking up a senior job at the Commonwealth Laboratories in Boston.

Anna O'Connell has been at FCCC longer than anyone I know. She fulfilled the role of senior technician, but her contributions went far beyond what the title might imply. Anna was particularly good at introducing new techniques. Research depends on looking at problems in new ways, and, particularly in recent years, revolutionary new methods have sparked whole new fields. She was also the unofficial institutional memory of our group; she could remember the results of studies successful and not so successful, the people we collaborated with, the lives of our colleagues. For many years she was the total master of our collection of biological specimens and a firm guardian of their integrity. From time to time she would have to remind me that we were running out of storage space. I would reply with some inane remark such as "Something good will happen" or "God will provide," and Anna would set about using her own means to pry more room from the so-called Space Cadets—that is, functionaries of the FCCC administration charged with the awesome responsibility of resource allocation.

Appendix 2

Research on Hyaluronic Acid
(Oxford University, 1955)

HYALURONIC ACID, one of a large group of natural polysaccharides, is a long-chain carbohydrate polymer, with a disaccharide, beta-glucuronido-1-3 N-acetylglucosamine, constituting the repeating unit. Polymers are long thin chains of repeating chemical units. There are many natural polymers and many synthetics, such as the plastic fibers from which most of our clothing is now made. Hyaluronic acid is a constituent of the ground substance that permeates the connective tissue—the stuff between the cells—and is involved in ion transport, support, and storage. It is also found in the umbilical cord, the vitreous humor of the eye, and in joint fluid, where it is thought to impart unique lubricating properties.

In its native state in joint fluid, hyaluronic acid is always found with protein. We formulated the hypothesis that the protein is associated with the unique physical characteristics of the molecule, in particular its high viscosity that, it was thought, imparted essential lubricating characteristics. To test the hypothesis, we planned to treat the hyaluronic acid protein complex with an enzyme that would remove the protein. We would then compare the enzyme-treated material to the native complex to see whether there were any changes in the physical characteristics of the molecule. We used papain, a very powerful enzyme that attacks many proteins. It was originally extracted, as its name implies, from the fruit of the papaya tree. In the mid-1950s science was pretty much do-it-yourself, with few chemicals available from the science supply industry; the enzyme had to be prepared from its natural source. So we started with several papayas, from which I obtained the enzyme and double-crystallized it to ensure purity.

Physical measurements of the molecule, including viscosity and molecular weight, were made before and after treatment with the papain enzyme. The ultracentrifuge was a massive piece of machinery designed to spin solutions at ultra-high speeds to separate the molecules on the basis of their molecular weight and other characteristics. Ours was one of the original machines designed by the Swedish scientist Theodor Svedberg. It occupied an entire room in the basement of the biochemistry building, a space that reminded me of the engine room of the amphibious landing ship I had served on while I was in the Navy, with the exception that the machine was substantially more finicky than the diesels that propelled our ship. Because the rotor was subject to high speeds and gravitational forces, there was always the fear that it might explode and send pieces hurtling around the laboratory. The rotor was enclosed in a vessel made of the kind of armor plate steel that is used on battleships. Each run was an adventure.

The results were pretty clear-cut. The removal of the protein markedly changed the characteristics of the molecule, and the inference was that this might have some bearing on the pathology associated with chronic joint disease. Shortly after our research was published, there was a report from another laboratory that cast doubt on our results. It appeared that the enzyme we had used to remove the protein also had an effect on the long-chain sugars of hyaluronic acid. If that was the case, then our results, the changes in the physical characteristics of the molecule, could be a consequence not only of the removal of the protein but of the shortening of the sugar strands themselves. This was pretty disappointing; however, later work appeared to show that our overall conclusions were correct. The protein associated with the molecule in its natural state was central to its physical characteristics.

Appendix 3

The National Institutes of Health and the Funding of Basic Medical Research

DURING the 1960s and 1970s, the National Institutes of Health funded most of the basic research in biomedicine in the United States. This was in large part due to the interest of the general public in the furtherance of basic science and its application to medicine. The institutes that made up the National Institutes of Health were named for disease categories: Cancer, Heart, Arthritis and Metabolic Disease, Neurological Diseases, Infectious Disease, and so forth. However, the director of the NIH, the brilliant Dr. James A. Shannon, and his staff recognized the value of undirected research that did not have an apparent relevance to the disease for which the particular institute was named. The funding mechanisms encouraged initiative and imagination. The decisions on grant awards were made, not by government officials, but by committees of scientific peers from universities and research institutes, industry, and other sectors of the scientific community. Although the grants were made to an institution, the application emanated from an individual scientific investigator who determined the use of the funds. The administrations of the universities and the academic departments might exercise a certain measure of control, but each scientist, including junior scientists, could generate his or her own ideas and be responsible for his or her own research budget. In that sense, the system was entrepreneurial and avoided the situation in many foreign academic settings, where the directors of departments and institutes—or, as the Italians put it, the *Barone*—dominated research. This NIH system for scientific funding and variants of it have been credited with giving the United States its predominance in science after World War II.

The president of the Nobel Foundation, Professor Sune Bergstrom, commented on this democratization of science in the United States in an address he gave in 1976:

> [A]part from these basic economic prerequisites, there are other actors which have greatly contributed towards the rapidity of America's expansion in the research sector and which are perhaps of particular interest to Europeans. Universities all over the world expanded rapidly during the 1940s and 1950s. In many places, and not least in the European countries, this expansion took place with the retention of traditional hierarchic and inflexible structures.
>
> In the USA, on the other hand, the growth of university research was characterized by a dynamic openness in forms which might be characterized as a democracy of research workers. Many visitors to American institutions and scientific congresses after the war were struck by the natural way in which professors and students could conduct scientific discussions on a basis of equality and also by the practice of making young researchers responsible at an early stage in their careers for independent research projects within the big institutions.[1]

---

[1] *Le Prix Nobel en 1976* (Stockholm: Imprimerie Royale P. A. Norstedt & Soner, 1977), 17.

Appendix 4

Molecular Biology

HBV WAS the first human pathogenic virus to be sequenced. Part of the reason for this priority was that the HBV DNA chain is small, and total sequencing was feasible. A second reason was that HBV did not grow in tissue or organ culture, which had been considered necessary for an understanding of a virus's mechanisms. Sequencing was, among other things, a way to circumvent this disadvantage.

HBV DNA is circular and is made up of two parallel chains (see fig. 2, above). One of these chains is not complete in the mature virus. The HBV genome contains four genes,[1] S, C, P, and X; in the following paragraphs I will discuss functions of some of the products of these genes.

The S gene produces the surface antigen of the virus (HBsAg)— the protein that covers the whole virus—that we had originally called Australia antigen. It is actually made up of three proteins, pre-S1, pre-S2, and S, that are produced by different portions of the overall reading frame. HBsAg also makes up the small particles that do not contain DNA, do not replicate, are not infectious, and do not cause symptoms of disease. Most are circular, with a diameter of about twenty-four nanometers, but some are elongated tubelike

---

[1] Actually, they are called open reading frames (ORF); that is, a length of DNA sequences between a start signal (codon) for translation and a signal that stops translation. Translation is the step in the synthesis of proteins where the messenger RNA makes a string of amino acids, the building blocks of proteins.

structures of the same diameter as the circular particles but of varying length. These smaller particles make up the material that was extracted from the blood of HBV carriers to prepare the vaccine.

What is the function of the small HBsAg particles in the life history of the virus? One conjecture is that they defend HBV against the immune system of the host and allow it to infect the host for a long time. The ratio of the noninfectious small particles to whole virus particles is about 1000 to 1. If, as part of the host immune response to the infection, antibodies (or immune cellular reactions) are produced against HBsAg, then they will react with the small HBsAg particles, and the rare viral particles will be spared. This is a pretty clever mechanism that enables the virus to cause a long-term chronic infection and allows more time and opportunity for transmission to another person. Ironically, it was this elaborate protection scheme "devised" by HBV that resulted in the vaccine that has gone a long way toward the control of the virus.

In the 1980s several scientists and pharmaceutical companies were successful in cloning the HBsAg gene into *E. coli*, yeast, and other cells to produce surface antigen that was used to prepare the vaccine. By this technique, vast quantities of HBsAg are produced without the need to recruit carrier donors. One of the pioneers in this process was the Smith Kline pharmaceutical company, at the time headquartered in Philadelphia. Shortly after the procedure was introduced, I visited the new Smith Kline factory in Belgium purpose-built for the manufacture of the recombinant vaccine. The plant manager informed me that if they worked three full shifts, they could produce all the HBV vaccine required in the world! The HBV vaccine is one of the small number of commercially successful recombinant drugs currently in use and, at present, the only widely used human recombinant vaccine.

There was another important consequence of the introduction of the recombinant vaccine. The horror of the AIDS epidemic was becoming apparent just about the time that the blood-derived vaccine became widely available. There was an inordinate fear, particularly among health care personnel, of any products derived from blood, even though the process for extraction of the vaccine from the donor blood includes several steps—high temperature, low pH, the use of chemicals that denature live viruses—that would kill any known virus. A series of tests demonstrated that the vaccine was not contaminated, and animal testing also ensured that all live viruses were removed from the concoction. Despite the scientific evidence validating the safety of the product, there was some reluctance to use the vaccine. Although this attitude had an impact in the United States, it did not, apparently, slow the vaccination programs in Asia, where the great fear of liver disease and primary cancer of the liver impelled the program forward.

The C gene produces two proteins. The "core antigen" (HBcAg) is the smaller protein. The "e-antigen" (HBeAg) is larger and consists of HBcAg plus an additional small piece produced by the pre-core region of the C gene. (I know the nomenclature is a little confusing, but hang in.) HBcAg provides a circular cover for the DNA and the RNA that are produced at different times in the replication cycle. HBeAg is exported from the liver cell, where it is produced, and enters the sera of infected individuals in whom the virus is actively replicating. HBeAg in the serum is an indication that there is active disease, and that the individual is infectious. An antibody against HBeAg (anti-HBeAg) is present in the blood when the replication activity slows down or stops. Its presence can be a sign of recovery and is used as a measure of the effectiveness of treatment for HBV infection.

The HBeAg marker proved very useful early in the vaccination program when vaccine was scarce and available only for those at highest risk. Pregnant women who are carriers of the virus, and who also have HBeAg, are much more likely to transmit virus to their newborns than pregnant women–carriers who do not, or women who are not carriers at all. In the early stages of the vaccination program in Taiwan and Japan, all pregnant women were tested for HBsAg and, if they were positive, for HBeAg. If they were positive for the latter, then their newborns were top priority candidates for vaccination. As the vaccine became more available, all newborns were vaccinated independent of the mother's status. But in some programs testing of mothers for HBsAg and HBeAg still continues.

If the mother is found to be HBeAg-positive, as an added precaution the child is given immune globulin that contains a large amount of the anti-HBs in addition to the vaccine. The immune globulin acts immediately, and the vaccine acts later when the host itself provides the immune response. However, clinical studies have shown that, in practice, using both the immune globulin and the vaccine is not much better than administering the vaccine by itself. Most vaccination programs simply provide the vaccine to all newborns.

One of the reasons I have gone into detail concerning the e-antigen is the fascinating question as to why the virus produces HBcAg, which stays in the cell, and the nearly similar but slightly larger HBeAg, which gets into the blood and elsewhere in the body. Surely the virus—or evolution, or Nature, or whatever "designs" viruses— did not develop this mechanism to facilitate the manufacture of diagnostic tests for clinicians and epidemiologists. What are the conjectures[2] concerning this phenomenon?

Professor Howard Thomas at St. Mary's Hospital in London has offered an interesting possible explanation. The pathology caused by HBV does not appear to be a consequence of the direct action of the virus on the cell. The culprit is the host cellular immune response to HBcAg and, probably, HBsAg, present on the liver cells. HBeAg has a great deal of common antigenicity with HBcAg because many of the peptides are identical. If it enters the blood early in infection or in utero when the conceptus is exposed to its mother's blood, then the newborn would become tolerant to HBeAg *and* HBcAg. In later life, when large amounts of HBcAg are expressed in the infected liver cells, the host immune response would be blunted by its tolerant state and would be less effective in destroying the cells and eliminating the virus. If true, this is another clever technique for maintaining the virus in its host for decades and increasing its probability of transmission to others. Not bad for a lowly virus. I doubt that I would have thought of it if the virus had not inspired the idea!

---

[2] A conjecture is really a hypothesis, but one devised when there are few data to constrain the imagination.

The Region P is the largest gene and overlaps all three of the others. It codes for several functions, including the enzymes that are necessary for the replication of the virus, the DNA polymerase and reverse transcriptase. Region X is the last of the open reading frames. When it was first identified, its function was not known, and the mystery letter X was used as the designator. Its function is still unclear, but not for lack of investigative effort. The protein product of the gene, HBxAg, appears to activate the transcription of the HBV genes and also other genes in the host cells. This could mean that protein products of the virus could have an effect on cellular functions of the host not directly related to the apparent "goals" of the virus, an interesting area for exploration. There is also experimental evidence that the gene or its product may be carcinogenic—that is, it is one of the agents brought into the host by the virus that may actually cause cancer. This is still an unsettled question but could provide an avenue for the development of anticancer agents.

I will briefly summarize the state of play in the understanding of the molecular biology of HBV and primary cancer of the liver. The DNA of HBV is integrated into the liver cell DNA of patients with hepatocellular carcinoma (HCC). It may also be integrated into the liver cells of carriers and, presumably, precedes cancer. The integration is not of the whole HBV genome but rather of bits and pieces; parts of the S and X genes are usually found, but C gene fragments are not. In humans, integration does not consistently favor a particular site, but it is not haphazardly random. There are favored sites for integration—for example, a narrow piece that includes the region called DR-1 located at one end of the more or less complete negative DNA strand. In humans, the integration sites are not systematically associated with genes that are associated with the ongoing process of cancer(oncogenes). They also do not bear a consistent direct relation to tumor suppressor genes ("antioncogenes").

There are chromosomal and other changes in patients with HCC that do not appear to be directly related to HBV but could result from its presence in the cells. These include chromosomal losses that may be a consequence of the ongoing cancer process. There are mutations in the *p53* gene and loss of tumor suppressor genes, changes often seen in cancers. These do not appear to be very specific. It is as if the presence of the virus shakes up the host's genome and chromosomes in some not easily predictable but not totally random manner. Gradually, the molecular biology of HCC is being worked out, all the while revealing possible sites for therapeutic and preventive intervention. The remarkable tools of molecular biology and the inexhaustible optimism of its practitioners will eventually result in a satisfactory and, undoubtedly, complicated explanation of carcinogenesis.

Appendix 5

A Gazetteer of Selected Place-Names Used in the Text

Place	Country	Comments
Afragola	Italy	Provincial city near Naples
Albina	Suriname	Town on the Marowijne R.
Anaktuvuk Pass	AK, USA	Remote Inuit community in Brooks Range
Babraham	UK	Site of research station, near Cambridge
Banjul	The Gambia	Capital city, formerly Bathurst
Barrow	AK, USA	Town on the Arctic Ocean littoral; site of Arctic Research Lab, Office of Naval Research
Belem	Brazil	City at the mouths of the Amazon
Bida	Nigeria	Inland region
Bratislava	Czechoslovakia (former)	Major city on the Danube
Brooks Range	AK, USA	Mountain range in the north
Cebu	Philippines	Island where family studies on Au were conducted
Chi-tung County	PRC	North shore of Yangtze R. across from Shanghai
Cottica R.	Suriname	Major river in north
Cumae	Italy	Ancient Greek colony near Naples
Dakar	Senegal	Capital city
Doonerak Mtn.	AK, USA	Highest peak in the Brooks Range
Dutch Guiana	S. America	Name for Suriname during the colonial period
Eniwetok	Marshall Islands	Large atoll in the former US Trust Territories of the Pacific Islands

Place	Country	Comments
Entebbe	Uganda	Major city
Fairbanks	AK, USA	Largest city in the north; site of Ladd Air Force Base
Fox Chase	PA, USA	Neighborhood in the north of Philadelphia; site of Fox Chase Cancer Center
French Guiana	S. America	French colony east of Suriname
Guipuzco	Spain	Northern province in the Basque area
Ibadan	Nigeria	Principal city of the western region
Jos	Nigeria	Major city on the Jos Plateau
Kaduna	Nigeria	Major city in the north
Kampala	Uganda	Capital and major city
Knossos	Crete, Greece	Seat of King Minos and Queen Pasiphae
Lagos	Nigeria	Former capital
Langatabatje	Suriname	Island capital of the Paramaccaners, Marowijne R.
Luzon	Philippines	Main island in the north of the island nation
Macedonia	Greece	Northern province, adjacent to the contemporary Republic of Macedonia
Mali	Africa	Inland country to the east of Senegal
Marowijne District	Suriname	Location of Moengo and Albina
Marshall Islands	Central Pacific	Former US Trust Territory
Moengo	Suriname	Aluminum-mining town on the Cottica R.
Moluccas	Indonesia	Group of islands
Netherlands East Indies	Pacific	Former colony of the Netherlands; now Republic of Indonesia
Pankshin	Nigeria	Provincial center on the Jos Plateau
Paramaribo	Suriname	Capital and port
Perth	Australia	Capital; major city of Western Australia
Recife	Brazil	Major city on the east coast
Sabah	Malaysia	On the island of Borneo
San Sebastian	Spain	Major city of Guipuzco
Santa Cruz Mtns.	CA, USA	Chain of mountains and hills stretching south from San Francisco ("The Coast Range")
Sea Islands	SC and GA, USA	Series of low island off the Atlantic coast of SC and GA
Senegal	Africa	Westernmost country in Africa
Siena	Italy	Major city in the north
Taipei	Taiwan	Major city of the island
Ternate	Indonesia	Located in the Moluccas, Indonesia
Titan	Saturn	A moon

Place	Country	Comments
Trinidad	Caribbean	An island nation along with Tobago
Turku	Finland	Major city of the west
Visayan Islands	Philippines	Cebu is in this group of islands
Vom	Nigeria	On the Jos plateau; site of the trypanosome research station
Wainwright	AK, USA	Inuit community on the Bering Sea; site of field trip

Index

Page references followed by *fig* indicate figures.